Epidemiology of Injury in Adventure and Extreme Sports

# Medicine and Sport Science

## Vol. 58

# Epidemiology of Injury in Adventure and Extreme Sports

Volume Editors

Travis W. Heggie Bowling Green, Ohio
Dennis J. Caine Grand Forks, N. Dak.

18 figures and 46 tables, 2012

KARGER Basel · Freiburg · Paris · London · New York · New Delhi · Bangkok · Beijing · Tokyo · Kuala Lumpur · Singapore · Sydney

**Medicine and Sport Science**
Founded 1968 by E. Jokl, Lexington, Ky.

**Travis W. Heggie, PhD**
Division of Sport Management
Recreation and Tourism
Bowling Green State University
Bowling Green, OH 43403 (USA)

**Dennis J. Caine, PhD**
Department of Physical Education
Exercise Science and Wellness
Hyslop Sports Center
University of North Dakota
Grand Forks, ND 58202-8235 (USA)

Library of Congress Cataloging-in-Publication Data

Epidemiology of injury in adventure and extreme sports / volume editors, Travis W. Heggie, Dennis J. Caine.
p. ; cm. -- (Medicine and sport science, ISSN 0254-5020 ; v. 58)
Includes bibliographical references and index.
ISBN 978-3-318-02164-6 (hard cover : alk. paper) -- ISBN 978-3-318-02165-3 (e-ISBN)
I. Heggie, Travis W. II. Caine, Dennis John, 1949- III. Series: Medicine and sport science ; v. 58. 0254-5020
[DNLM: 1. Athletic Injuries--epidemiology. 2. Sports. W1 ME649Q v.58 2012 / QT 261]

617.1'027--dc23

2012018992

Bibliographic Indices. This publication is listed in bibliographic services, including Current Contents®.


www.karger.com
Printed in Switzerland on acid-free and non-aging paper (ISO 9706) by Kraft Druck GmbH, Ettlingen
ISSN 0254–5020
e-ISSN 1662–2812
ISBN 978–3–318–02164–6
e-ISBN 978–3–318–02165–3

# Contents

Heggie TW, Caine DJ (eds): Epidemiology of Injury in Adventure and Extreme Sports.
Med Sport Sci. Basel, Karger, 2012, vol 58, pp 1–16

# The Epidemiology of Injury in Adventure and Extreme Sports

Dennis J. Caine

Department of Physical Education, Exercise Science and Wellness, University of North Dakota, Grand Forks, N. Dak., USA

**Abstract**

The objective of this article is to provide an overview of the current knowledge related to the epidemiology of injury in selected adventure and extreme sports. PubMed and Google Scholar were searched using the terms 'epidemiology', 'injury,' 'adventure sports' and 'extreme sports'. Publications from the past 10 years were largely selected, but commonly referenced or highly regarded older publications were also included. References lists of articles identified in the search strategy were also searched and articles selected that were judged to be relevant. Important aspects of the epidemiology of injury related to adventure and extreme sports are discussed including occurrence of injury, who is affected by injury, where and when injury occurs, injury outcome, risk factors, inciting events, prevention and further research. Given the life-changing impact injury can have in sports (personal, social, financial, psychological, political, and medical), the current paucity of well-designed descriptive and particularly analytical epidemiological studies in some adventure and extreme sports is disturbing. The importance of denominator-based and longitudinal data collection in obtaining an accurate picture of injury risk and severity and as a basis for testing risk factors and evaluating preventive measures is emphasized. 

It is difficult to determine exactly when adventure and extreme sports came to refer to a growing group of popular modern sports. However, there is little question that their rise in popularity has been nothing short of phenomenal. Different schools of thought tie the origin of adventure and extreme sports to the ancient Hawaiian sport of surfing or the countercultural movements of the 1960s. Others suggest that the popularity of these sports is simply the reaction to the increased safety of modern life, enhanced sports technology, and exceptional media marketing. Regardless of which school of thought one follows, adventure and extreme sport activities are now broadly defined as individualistic sports containing structural components of real or perceived danger [1]. These activities often involve speed, height, a high level of physical exertion, and highly specialized gear or spectacular stunts. Moreover, participants in

**Table 1.** SGMA Sports and Fitness Participation Report, 2011

| Sport activity | Number of participants (participated at least once in 2010) |
|---|---|
| Bicycling* (BMX) | 2,369,000 |
| Bicycling (mountain) | 7,161,000 |
| Backpacking (overnight) | 8,439,000 |
| Boardsailing/windsurfing* | 1,617,000 |
| Canoeing | 10,553,000 |
| Climbing* | 2,198,000 |
| Hiking | 32,496,000 |
| Jet ski | 7,753,000 |
| Kayaking* (recreational, sea, whitewater) | 10,451,000 |
| Rafting | 4,460,000 |
| Scuba diving* | 3,153,000 |
| Surfing | 2,276,000 |
| Wakeboarding | 3,645,000 |

* Sports which have shown a 20% or greater increase in number of participants from 2009 to 2010.

these activities often compete in variable environmental conditions such as those that are weather- and-terrain related, including wind, snow, water and mountains [2].

Media coverage of adventure and extreme sports events has increased considerably in recent years to the point that US sports broadcaster ESPN broadcasts the ever popular 'X Games' on an annual basis. This event, along with former events such as the 'Gravity Games' and the 'Gorge Games' have included rollerblading, skateboarding, snowboarding, windsurfing, kiteboarding, BMX, and motocross into their definition of extreme sports. Other sources have included sports such as motorcycle racing, rock climbing, and base jumping in their definitions. This all points to the fact that adventure and extreme sports are not just a fad. Instead, due to the media attention that these sports are receiving, they are becoming ever more popular with youth and young adults. For example, according to the Sporting Goods Manufacturing Association (SGMA) analysis of the Sports and Fitness Participation Report (2011 edition), extreme sports are an appealing recreational and athletic option for millions of Americans [3]. The most popular adventure and extreme sports in the USA during 2010 (6 years of age or older) are listed in table 1.

There is now overwhelming evidence that regular physical activity has important and wide-ranging health benefits ranging from reduced risk of chronic diseases such as heart disease, type 2 diabetes, and some cancers to enhanced function and preservation of function with age [4]. There is concern, however, whether the health benefits of sports participation outweigh the risk of injury and long-term disability [5]. By their very nature, participation in adventure and extreme sports involves performance

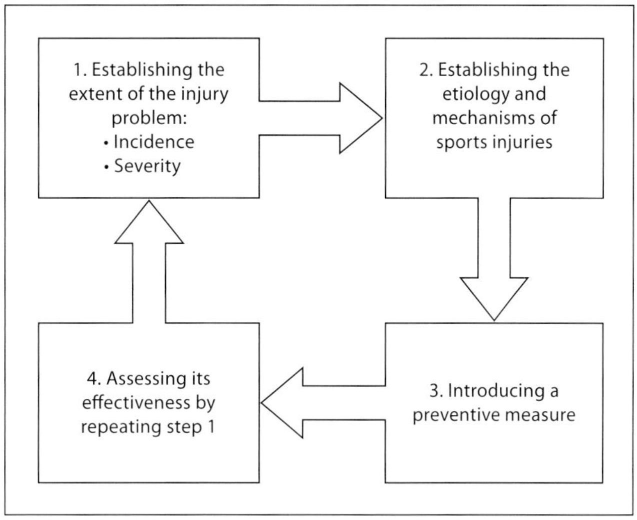


**Fig. 1.** Four-step sequence of injury prevention research. Reproduced from van Mechelen et al. [6] with permission from Springer Healthcare/Adis Data Information BV.

in variable and often unpredictable environmental conditions that may be associated with significant physical risks.

Participants in adventure and extreme sports and everyone who works with them, whether they are parents, sports medicine personnel, sports governing bodies, or coaches, need to know answers to questions such as: Is the risk of injury greater in some sport activities, or level of activities, than in others? Where are injuries most likely to occur, both in terms of anatomic and environmental location? What is the outcome of injury, including in terms of types, severity, and cost? Are some physical, psychological, or sport-related factors associated with an increased risk of injury? How effective are the preventive measures that have been implemented? These are all questions which need to be answered through scientific investigation. Providing this information is an important objective of epidemiological research related to adventure and extreme sports.

## The Epidemiological Approach

Injury epidemiology is the study of the distribution and determinants of varying rates of injuries in human populations for the purpose of identifying and implementing measures to prevent their development and spread. A model outlining the epidemiologic approach to sports injury prevention was first proposed by van Mechelen et al. [6] (fig. 1). Sports injury prevention research involves a sequence of prevention [6]. First, research establishes the extent of injury, including both incidence and severity. Second, research explores its etiology (i.e., the causes and implications of injury). Third, research creates a prevention strategy to reduce the injury burden.

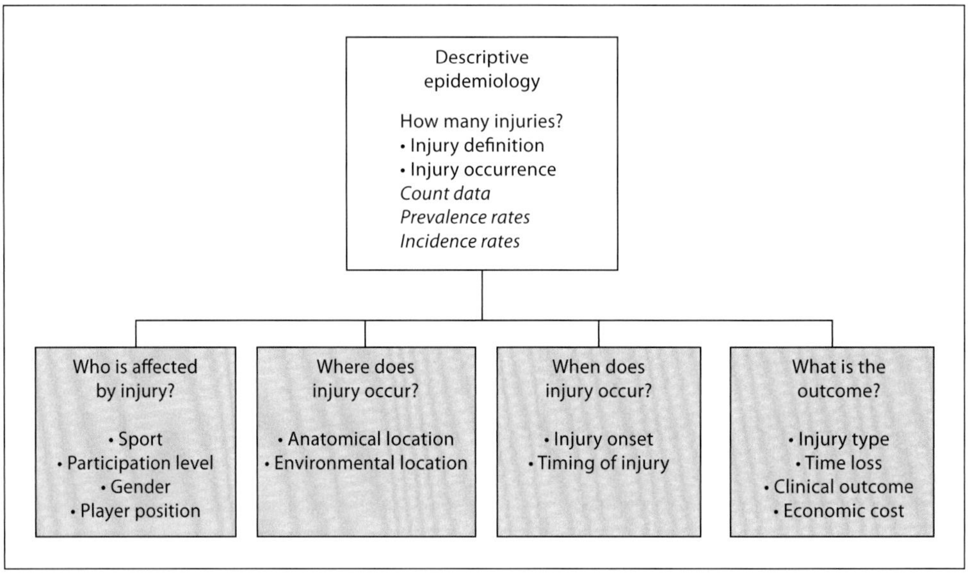


**Fig. 2.** Descriptive epidemiology of sports injuries. Reproduced from Caine et al. [9] with permission from Wolters Kluwer Health.

Last, research evaluates the effectiveness of the implemented prevention strategy by re-examining the extent of injury.

The epidemiologist in sports medicine is concerned with quantifying injury occurrence *(how much)* with respect to *who* is affected by injury, *where* and *when* injuries occur, and *what* is their outcome (step 1), for the purpose of explaining *why* and *how* injuries occur (step 2) and identifying strategies to control and prevent them (steps 3 and 4) [7]. The study of the distribution of varying rates of injuries (i.e., who, where, when, what) is referred to as descriptive epidemiology. The study of the determinants of an exhibited distribution of varying rates of injuries (i.e., why and how) and the identification and implementation of preventive strategies is referred to as analytical epidemiology [8].

## Descriptive Epidemiology

Descriptive epidemiology is by far the most common type of epidemiologic research that has been published in the adventure and extreme sports injury literature and arises from observational research, including case series, cross-sectional, and cohort studies. A diagram illustrating important aspects of the descriptive epidemiology of sports-related injuries is shown in figure 2 [9]. These components are discussed below with the purpose of highlighting their various contributions to understanding the distribution of adventure and extreme sport injuries.

In descriptive epidemiology the researcher attempts to quantify the occurrence of injury. The most basic measure of injury occurrence is a simple count of injured persons or fatalities. For example, Rekand et al. [10] reported on 9 patients with spinal cord injury caused by paragliding accidents. The data were obtained from hospital files at all three spinal units in Norway and cross-checked with the Norwegian Paragliding Association's voluntary registry for injuries. Count data are also used to report fatalities related to participation in extreme and adventure sports. For example, Garland [11] reported that in the USA during 1982–2010, there were 11,001 deaths related to all-terrain vehicle use. Twenty-five percent (2,775) of these fatalities involved children younger than 16 years of age.

In order to investigate the rate and distribution of injuries it is necessary to know the size of the source population from which the injured individuals were derived, or the population at risk. The two most commonly reported rates in the sports injury literature are *incidence* and *prevalence*. Prevalence pertains to the total number of cases, new or old, that exist in a population at risk at a specific period of time. This can be at a certain point of time (point prevalence) or during a time period (period prevalence) [12]. An example of a prevalence rate published in the adventure and extreme sport injury literature is percent rates for specific conditions such as radiographic changes in the hands and fingers of 12 young, high-level climbers [13]. A limitation of prevalence data is that only injuries present during the time of the survey period are registered, thus data are not necessarily representative of all injuries in a population.

The two types of injury incidence most commonly reported in the sports injury literature are clinical incidence and incidence rates. *Clinical incidence* refers to the number of incident injuries divided by the total number of athletes at risk and usually multiplied by some *k* value (e.g., 100) [14]. For example, Wilmshurst et al. [15] reported 22 cases of decompression illness per 10,000 amateur scuba divers per year. Similarly, Hart et al. [16] reported 0.3 deaths per 10,000 divers in a report of scuba diving accidents in Leicester, UK, over a period of 5 years.

Clinical incidence may serve as an indication of clinical or resource utilization; however, it does not account for the potential variance in exposure of participants to risk of injury [14]. For example, divers may be differentially exposed to risk of injury because of varying numbers of dives per year.

*Incidence rate* refers to the number of incident injuries divided by the total time-at-risk and usually multiplied by some *k* value (e.g., 1,000) [14]. It is the preferred measure of incidence in research studies because it can accommodate variations in exposure time of individual participants. Different units of time-at-risk, varying in precision, have been used to calculate incidence rates in recent literature adventure and extreme sports literature. These include reporting the number of injuries per *k* time exposures (one time exposure is typically defined as 1 individual participating in 1 h of activity in which there is the possibility of sustaining a sport-related injury) and per *k* element exposures (one element exposure is defined as 1 individual participating in one element of activity in which there is the possibility of sustaining an athletic injury). For example, Neuhof et al. [17] reported an acute injury rate of 0.2 per 1,000 h sport performance in 1,962 sport climbers. Examples of exposure elements common in adventure and extreme sports include climbs, summits, surfer days, personal watercrafts in operation, (scuba) dives, and (base) jumps. For example, Taylor et al. [18] reported a rate of 2.2 injuries per 1,000 surfer days among 646 recreational surfers.

A difficulty that may arise in comparing incidence rates from different studies relates to the injury definition employed. A review of the adventure and extreme sports literature reveals that few common operational definitions exist for injury. Definitions include such criteria as presence of a new symptom or complaint, decreased function of a body part or decreased athletic performance, cessation of practice or competition activities, and consultation with medical or training personnel. Clearly, if injury is defined differently across studies, a meaningful comparison of injury rates is compromised due to different criteria for determining numerator values. Notably, representatives of several international sport organizations recently published methodological consensus statements that identify definitions and methodology to ensure consistency and comparability of results in studies examining injury in their sports [19–21].

*Who Is Affected by Injury?*

As might be expected, injury rates are most often categorized according to sport participation (e.g., mountaineering, sport climbing, ice climbing) and the way in which participants are organized for sports (e.g., recreational or competitive). In addition to participation level, injury rates are also reported relative to age and gender. Given the variance in injury definitions across studies, perhaps the most reliable within- or across-sport comparisons arise from those studies which use a common, exposure-based injury definition and surveillance protocol monitored by health professionals. However, most data on adventure and extreme sports arise from hospital and emergency room data, trauma registries, national injury registries, sport associations and commissions, emergency services, and search and rescue reports. As a result, reliable denominator data and therefore determination of incidence rates are often absent from injury reports.

*Where Does Injury Occur?*

Determination of 'where' injury occurs involves identification of the anatomical and environmental locations of injury. Anatomical locations include body region of injury (e.g., upper extremity) as well as specific body parts (e.g., shoulder, ankle). Identification of commonly injured anatomical locations alerts healthcare personnel to injury sites in need of special attention, for example during pre-participation musculoskeletal assessment. Information on high injury risk locations also provides important 'targets' for preventive measures. For example, a common injury associated with skydiving is ankle injury incurred during landing. Parachute ankle braces were subsequently developed and have been shown to reduce frequency of parachute ankle injuries by about half [22].

Environmental location provides information on the distribution of injury by where in the environment or setting the injury occurred. This information alerts healthcare professional to environmental situations which may be associated with an elevated risk injury. Environmental locations reported in the adventure and extreme sports injury literature include surface or terrain on which the activity takes place, for example indoor or outdoor climbing or grade of terrain associated with mountaineering; geographical location, for example public areas versus skate parks for skateboarders; proximity to others or obstacles (e.g., overcrowding among personal watercraft riders), and whether the injury occurred in practice or competition. Information on high-risk settings is of course useful in identifying important targets for further study, including application of preventive measures.

Most research on environmental location report distribution of environmental factors as frequency or percent values. However, the importance of providing both types of information – percent values and incidences rates – is perhaps best underscored by comparisons of injury between practice and competition. For many sports, the proportion of injuries incurred in practice is much greater than for competition, most likely because much more time is spent in practice than competition. However, when incidence rates are compared, the common finding is a higher injury incidence in competition in many sports. Competitors are much more likely to be participating at greater intensity and speeds in competition and tournaments than in practice, thus increasing the risk of sustaining an injury.

*When Does Injury Occur?*

As figure 2 indicates, the next characteristic of injury distribution is the *when* of injury occurrence. Time factors are typically expressed in terms of injury onset and time of injury. There are two broad categories of injury onset that differ markedly in their etiology. Injuries that occur suddenly are often termed acute or sudden impact injuries and are usually the result of a single, traumatic event. Common examples include wrist fractures, ankle sprains, shoulder dislocations, and hamstring muscle strain. Overuse injuries are more subtle and develop gradually over time. They are the result of repetitive microtrauma to the tendons, bones and joints. An example of a common overuse injury common among sport climbers is epicondylitis and tenosynovitis of the finger flexor tendons [23]. An injury history may actually involve both categories of injury onset, such as when an acute injury is superimposed on a chronic mechanism.

Most epidemiological studies of injury in the adventure and extreme sports injury literature do not distinguish between acute and overuse injuries. However, this is an important oversight, particularly in studies that analyze risk factors since risk factors for overuse and acute injuries are not necessarily the same. The importance of identifying injury onset is also important given the growing evidence of overuse problems in sport, particularly among child and adolescent participants. Information on incidence of overuse injury is important if we are to fully comprehend the impact of these injuries and the role of injury countermeasures.

Examples of timing of injury include time into practice, time of day, and time of season or year when injury occurs. It stands to reason that if rates are higher during a particular time period, then efforts to better understand the risk factors for the elevated risk are in order and appropriate preventive measures should be applied to reduce risk during this time. For example, if the proportion of injuries is shown to be greater during the latter part of a competition or event, then fatigue could be considered as a possible contributing factor [24].

### *What Is the Outcome?*

Injury outcome can span a broad spectrum from abrasions to fractures, to those injuries that result in severe permanent functional disability (i.e., catastrophic injuries) or even death. In the epidemiologic literature on sports injuries injury severity is typically indicated by one or more of the following: injury type, time loss, residual symptoms, and economics costs. Assessment in each of these areas is important to quantification of the extent of the injury problem. It may be, for example, that injury incidence is similar in two sports, however the type and severity of injury may vary considerably between these sports.

#### Injury Type

Identification of common injury types is important because it alerts sports medicine personnel to injury types in need of special attention and it directs researchers in identifying and testing related risk factors and preventive measures. Most sports injury studies report injury types in general terms such as contusion or fracture, with few specifics on type of fracture, grade of injury and so forth. Injury types are generally reported as frequency or percent values. However, studies should also provide incidence rate values, particularly for specific injury types such as concussion. This latter approach facilitates analysis of risk factors and preventive measures related to these injury types.

#### Injury Severity

A useful measure of injury severity and one often used in the literature on sports injuries is the duration of restriction from athletic performance subsequent to injury. Some studies reporting time loss use total or average number of days lost from practice, competition, or from work as a measure of injury severity. Although the use of days lost from participation may be among the more precise representations of injury severity in the literature, this approach is not without problems. For example, subjective factors, such as personal motivation, peer influence, or coaching staff reluctance/

encouragement, may determine if and when players return to play. Accessibility to a healthcare professional and location of injury may also impact decision of when to return to participation.

In addition to length of hospital admission and level of care required, a number of hospital studies of injury related to adventure and extreme sports have used objective scoring systems of injury severity. For example, Schöffl et al. [25] used the National Advisory Committee for Aeronautics (NACA) system for accidents in aviation to analyze injury and fatalities occurring in rick and ice climbing. Similarly, some studies have used the Injury Severity Score system (ISS) to describe injury severity. For example, Konkin at al. [26] reported a mean ISS of 10.5 in a population-based analysis of severe injuries from non-motorized wheeled vehicles (bicyclists, skateboarders, inline skaters). Similarly, Gorski et al. [27] used the ISS to describe severity of injuries associated with motocross accidents.

### Clinical Outcome

Clinical outcome includes such factors as re-injury, non-participation, residual effects, and fatalities. An unfortunate outcome of many injuries, at all levels of sport, is re-injury. It is believed that unresolved residual symptoms from previous injury predispose an athlete to recurrent injury at the same site [28]. Restricted joint motion leads to muscle atrophy and increased compensatory stress on other areas, thus predisposing to injury at other sites [29]. An athlete with previous injury who returns to participation is characterized by a changed injury risk profile, particularly if the original injury has not been properly rehabilitated. Unfortunately, few studies of adventure and extreme sports provide data related to the frequency or incidence of re-injury.

Perhaps the most important question one can ask related to injury severity relates to residual or the long-term effects of injury. However, with the exception of catastrophic injuries (including fatalities), surprisingly little is known about the long-term outcomes of adventure and extreme sport injuries, such as rates of post-traumatic osteoarthritis, sequalae of head injuries, and other trauma. The data on catastrophic injuries, like most injury data for adventure and extreme sports, arise primarily from hospital and emergency room data, trauma registries, national injury registries, sport associations and commissions (e.g., German Alpine Club, British Sub-Aqua Club), emergency services, and search and rescue reports. As a result, most of the data on catastrophic injuries, including fatalities, are count data. However, several studies provide clinical incidence or incidence rates for fatalities [16, 30].

### Economic Cost

Financial costs may be either direct or indirect. Direct costs are those incurred in conjunction with medical treatment (e.g., treatment, medication), and indirect costs are those associated with the loss of productivity because of increased morbidity and mortality levels. Although there have been several attempts to estimate these costs for a few selected sports and injury types, comparison of results has been hampered by differences in healthcare and wage compensation systems [31–34]. Studies need to show the economic impact of sports injuries on public resources in order to demonstrate the need for grants to support sports injury epidemiology research.

## Analytical Epidemiology

In the past, good descriptive data have led directly to suggestions for injury prevention that, once implemented, have helped to control and prevent the occurrence of severe sports and recreation injuries such as eye injuries in hockey (mandatory use of face shields) and spinal injuries in football (prohibition of head as first point of contact) [35]. However, although the institution of a preventive strategy on the basis of descriptive research has been shown to prevent injury, the most reliable suggestions for prevention are still believed to emerge from descriptive and analytical research where the extent of the injury problem (accounting for participation time), risk factors, and inciting factors have been established and where preventive measures have been tested through intervention studies [6, 36].

Analytical epidemiology focuses on *why* and *how* injuries occur (step 2) and identifying strategies to control and prevent them (steps 3 and 4). Analytical epidemiological research includes intervention studies or randomized control trials as well as cohort and case-control study designs. Cross-sectional designs have also been used to analyze risk factors. However, since cross-sectional studies are generally limited to data at one time point, they are unable to establish causality between exposures and the outcome because of lack of temporality in the study design.

In recent years there has been a promising and observable transition to research approaches etiologically rather than descriptively based to make participation safer for all participants. Preventive measures supported by research include ankle bracing, helmets, face shields, and the use of mouth guards [37]. Multiple interventions using warm-up, balance training, and neuromuscular control strategies have also been shown to be effective [37]. However, in the sports injury epidemiology literature on adventure and extreme sports, the approaches have been primarily descriptive-based, with few studies designed to test risk factors or to determine the effectiveness of preventive measures.

### *Risk Factors*

The epidemiological approach to sports injuries is rooted in the assumption that injuries do not happen purely by chance, so an important part of sports and recreation injury epidemiology is the identification of factors that contribute to the occurrence of injury. It should be understood, however, that this process is not an isolated one.

Risk factor analyses should be driven by a need to better understand the factors leading to injury in order to test and ultimately intervene with effective prevention strategies. Risk factors may be classified as intrinsic or extrinsic [38]. Intrinsic factors are individual biological and psychosocial characteristics predisposing a person to the outcome of injury such as previous injury, strength, or life stress. Once the athlete is 'predisposed', extrinsic or 'enabling' factors may facilitate manifestation of injury [39]. Extrinsic risk factors are factors that have an impact on the sport participant 'from without' and include such factors as coach's qualifications, playing time, and surface conditions. Risk factors can also be divided into modifiable and non-modifiable factors [40]. Modifiable risk factors refer to those that can be altered by injury prevention strategies to reduce injury rates. Although non-modifiable risk factors such as gender or age may be important considerations in many studies of injury prediction, it is above all important to study factors that are potentially modifiable. What complicates the identification and quantification of risks is that causality associated with injury is both extremely complex and dynamic in nature. In this regard, Meeuwisse et al. [41] proposed a dynamic recursive model that accommodates a multifactorial assessment of causation in sport injuries and emphasizes the fact that adaptations occur within the context of repeated participation in sport (both in the presence and absence of injury) that alter risk and affect etiology in a dynamic, recursive fashion (see fig. 3) [41]. According to the dynamic recursive model, both intrinsic and extrinsic risk factors are subject to change in the context of repeated participation in sport. For example, if an injury does occur, the athlete may be removed from participation if they do not fully recover. However, some degree of recovery may allow the athlete to return to participation and, therefore repeat participation. Adaptations in the athlete may also occur due to participation itself in the absence of injury, thus also modifying risk factors [42].

Analysis of sports injury risk factors has produced a number of significant injury predictors – including such factors as age, gender (specific to sport and type of injury), previous injury, and stressful life events – which have shown consistent results across multiple studies [29]. As mentioned above, the literature on risk factors is rather limited for adventure and extreme sports. However, risk factors which have been the focus of attention in some of this literature include personality traits related to risk-taking, body mass index, age, experience, exposure, self-efficacy, equipment, level of task difficulty, technique, education, inadequate physical condition, wearing of safety equipment failure, engine size, not being certified, and environmental conditions (e.g., size of waves, speed of water, strong or turbulent winds).

Much of the risk factor literature in adventure and extreme sports is characterized by one or more of the following limitations: injury definitions and methods of injury data collection are variable; incidence rates based on clinical incidence rather than incidence rates (i.e., rates based on hours or sessions of exposure), and inappropriate analyses for detecting multifactorial risks. As a result, much of this research should be viewed as initial work in the important search for injury

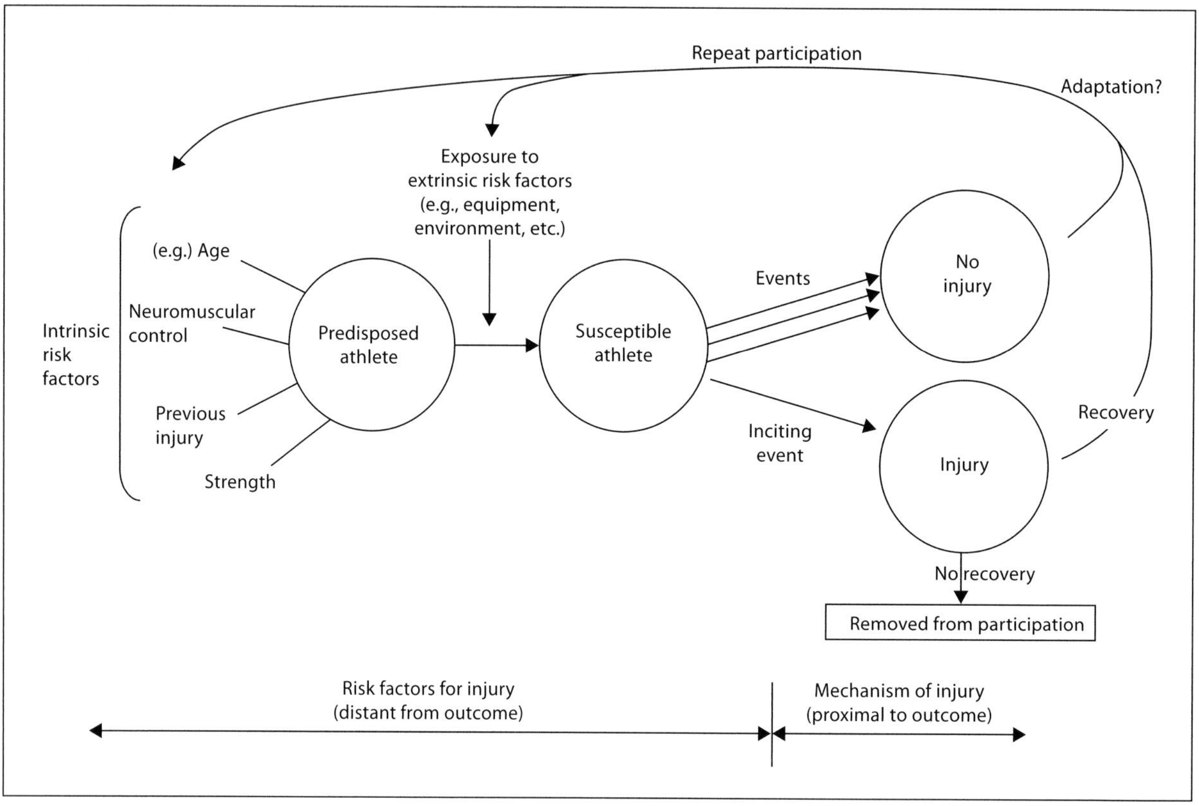


**Fig. 3.** Recursive model of etiology in sport injury. Reproduced from Meeuwisse et al. [41] with permission from Wolters Kluwer Health.

predictors and that may provide interesting variables for manipulation in other study designs.

*Inciting Events*

Although risk factors may render the sport participant more susceptible to injury, they are not usually sufficient for an injury to occur. Meeuwisse [39] suggests that the final element in the web of causation involves an inciting event (see fig. 3). Although it is recognized that while sometimes an inciting event occurs to produce injury, more often events occur that result in no injury [42]. However, adaptations in the athlete may occur due to the participation itself (e.g., improved motor skill) [42]. An inciting event is more obviously (or visually) related to the injury than a risk factor and may be viewed as a precipitating factor associated with the definitive onset of injury. Inciting events may include the playing situation, player/opponent behavior, gross biomechanical description (whole body) and detailed biomechanical description (joint) [43]. Due to space restrictions, we encouraged authors of this volume to limit discussion of inciting events to actions or activities (situations) leading to injury. Examples of inciting events reported in the literature on injury in adventure and extreme sports including: falling, collision with stationary objects or others in the environment, rapid ascent and out-of-air (during scuba diving), vehicle rollovers, equipment failure, and awkward landings.

*Injury Prevention*

Once the analytical evidence points to an association between certain risk factors and injury, thereby establishing a degree of predictability for those participants who are likely to sustain injury, the next step in epidemiologic research is to seek ways to prevent or reduce the occurrence of such injury (i.e., steps 3 and 4, fig. 1). Testing the suggested preventive measure to determine its effectiveness is an important aspect of the analytical epidemiologic process and fulfills the ultimate goal of epidemiology – that is, prevention. Ideally, the effectiveness of injury prevention measures should be tested prior to recommending their general implementation.

The results of recent investigations of sports injury prevention strategies have been encouraging [37, 44]. For example, balance training appears to decrease the risk of lower extremity injuries, especially ankle injuries [45–49]. However, there has been very little research designed to determine the effectiveness of injury prevention measures in adventure and extreme sports. Most recommendations are intuitive with conclusions drawn from descriptive data; few studies have actually tested preventive measures. For example, protective headgear has been recommended for participants in several adventure and extreme sports [50–52]; however, with the exception of one study of the benefit of helmet-use in all-terrain vehicle trauma, the effect of this measure has not been studied [53]. Ethical, cost, and feasibility issues no doubt combine to preclude some types of experimental research.

## Further Research

Given the life-changing impact injury can have in sports (personal, social, financial, psychological, political, and medical), the current paucity of well-designed epidemiological studies in the majority of adventure and extreme sports is disturbing. Most adventure and extreme sports lack quality descriptive data, which provides the essential building block for analytical epidemiological studies. Few studies address injury risk factors and even fewer evaluate preventive measures. Major fundamental deficiencies identified in the chapter reviews of this book include inappropriate study designs, short data collection periods, inconsistent or poorly delineated definition(s) of reportable injury and failure to collect quality exposure data. The importance of denominator-based longitudinal data collection in obtaining an accurate picture of injury risk and severity and as a basis for testing risk factors and evaluating preventive measures cannot be overemphasized.

There is also an urgent need for sport governing bodies to provide incentive and guidance for epidemiological research. The recent publication of consensus statements on injury definitions and data collection procedures from two important international federations (Fédération Internationale de Football Association (FIFA) [19] and the International Rugby Board [20]), as well as the agreement statement of concussion arising from multiple international and national organizations [54], are significant steps in this process and provide models for other sport governing bodies to follow. And finally, there is a need for translational research to examine factors which impact the likelihood of a prevention strategy being adopted by the target population [55].

## References


1 Ewert AW, Hollenhorst SJ: Adventure recreation and its implications for wilderness. Int J Wilderness 1997;3:21–26.

2 Wikipedia: Extreme sport. Accessed March 16, 2011 at http://en.wikipedia.org/wiki/Extreme_sport

3 Sporting Good Manufacturer's Association (SGMA) Sports, Fitness & Recreational Activities Topline Participation Report 2011. Accessed January 2, 2012 at http://www.aahperd.org/naspe/advocacy/governmentRelations/upload/2011-SGMA-Participation-Topline-Report.pdf

4 Blair SN: Physical inactivity: the biggest public health problem in the 21st century. Br J Sports Med 2009;43:1–2.

5 Engebretsen L, Bahr R: Why is injury prevention in sports important? In Bahr R, Engebretsen L (eds): Sports Injury Prevention: Handbook of Sports Medicine. Oxford, Wiley-Blackwell, 2009, pp 1–6.

6 Van Mechelen W, Hlobil H, Kemper CG: Incidence, severity, aetiology and prevention of sport injuries. A review of concepts. Sports Med 1992;14:82–89.

7 Caine C, Caine D, Lindner K: The epidemiologic approach to sports injuries; in Caine C, Caine D, Lindner K (eds): Epidemiology of Sports Injuries. Champaign, Human Kinetics Publishers, 1996, pp 1–13.

8 Duncan DF: Epidemiology: Basis for Disease Prevention and Health Promotion. New York, MacMillan, 1988.

9 Caine D, Caine C, Maffulli N: Incidence and distribution of pediatric sport-related injuries. Clin J Sport Med 2006;16:501–514.

10 Rekand T, Schaaning EE, Varga V, Schattel U, Gronning M: Spinal Cord 2008;46:412–416.

11 Garland S: 2010 Annual Report of ATV-Related Deaths and Injuries: Consumer Product Safety Commission; 2010. Accessed on January 2, 2012 at http://www.cpsc.gov/library/foia/foia12/os/atv2010.pdf

12 Hebel JR, McCarter RJ: A Study Guide to Epidemiology and Biostatistics, ed 7. Sudbury, Jones & Bartlett, 2012.

13 Schöffl V, Hochholzer T, Imhoff A: Radiographic changes in the hands and fingers of young, high-level climbers. Am J Sports Med 2004;32:1688–1694.

14 Knowles SB, Marshall SW, Guskiewicz KM: Issues in estimating risks and rates in sports injury research. J Athl Train 2006;41:207–215.

15 Wilmshurst PT, Allen A, Parish T: Incidence of decompression illness in amateur scuba divers. Health Trends 1994;26:116–118

16 Hart AJ, White SA, Conboy PJ, Bodiwala G, Quinton D: Open water scuba diving accidents at Leicester: five years' experience. J Accid Emerg Med 1999; 16:198–200.

17 Neuhof A, Hennig FF, Schoffl I, Schoffl V: Injury risk evaluation in sport climbing. Int J Sports Med 2011;32:794–800.

18 Taylor KS, Zoltan TB, Achar SA: Medical illnesses and injuries encountered during surfing. Curr Sports Med Rep 2006;5:262–267.

19 Fuller C, Ekstrand J, Junge A, Andersen T, Bahr R, Dvorak J, Hägglund M, McCrory P, Meeuwisse W: Consensus statement on injury definitions and data collection procedures in studies of football (soccer) injuries. Br J Sports Med 2006;40:193–201.

20 Fuller C, Molloy M, Bagate C, Bahr R, Brooks J, Donson H, Kemp S, McCrory P, McIntosh A, Meeuwisse W, Quarrie K, Raftery M, Wiley P: Consensus statement on injury definitions and data collection procedures for studies of injuries in rugby union. Clin J Sports Med 2007;17:177–181.

21 Schöffl V, Morrison AB, Hefti U, Schwarz U, Kupper T: The UIAA Medical Commission Injury Classification for Mountaineering and Climbing Sports; in No 17.10.05.2010 ed. Bern, Official Standards of the Union Internationale des Associations d'Alpinisme (UIAA), 2010, pp 1–8.

22 Knapik JJ, Spiess A, Swedler DI, et al: Systematic review of the parachute ankle brace: injury risk reduction and cost effectiveness. Am J Prev Med 2010;38:S181–S188.

23 Schöffl V, Hochholzer T, Winkelmann HP, Strecker W: Differential diagnosis of finger pain in sport climbers. Dtsch Z Sportmed 2003;54:38–43.

24 Caine D: Epidemiology of sports injuries; in Micheli L (ed): Encyclopedia of Sports Medicine. New York, Sage, 2011, vol 2, pp 432–440.

25 Schöffl V, Morrison AB, Schwarz U, Schöffl I, Kuppter T: Evaluation of injury and fatality risk in rock and ice climbing sport. Sport Med 2010;40: 657–659.

26 Konkin DE, Garraway N, Hameed SM, Brown DR, Granger R, Wheeler S, Simons RK: Population-based analysis of severe injuries from non-motorized wheeled vehicles. Am J Surg 2006;19:615–618.

27 Gorski TF, Gorski YC, McLeod G, Suh D, Cordero R, Essien F, Berry D, Dada F: Patterns of injury and outcomes associated with motocross accidents. Am Surg 2003;69:895–898.

28 Rauh MJ, Margherita AJ, Rice SG, et al: High school cross-country running injuries: a longitudinal study. Clin J Sport Med 2000;10:110–116.

29 Caine D, Maffulli N, Caine C: Epidemiology of injury in child and adolescent sports: injury rates, risk factors, and prevention. Clin Sports Med 2008; 27:19–50.

30 Schussmann LC, Lutz LJ, Shaw RR, Bohn CR: The epidemiology of mountaineering and rock climbing accidents. Wilderness Environ Med 1990;1:235–248.

31 Bentley TA, Page SJ, Macky KA: Adventure tourism and adventure sports injury: the New Zealand experience. Appl Ergon 2007;38:791–796.

32 Lee CT, Williams P, Hadden WA: Parachuting for charity: is it worth the money? A 5-year audit of parachute injuries in Tayside and the cost to the NHS. Injury 1999;30:283–287.

33 Macdonald DJ, McGlone S, Exton A, Perry S: A new skatepark: the impact on the local hospital emergency. Injury 2006;37:238–242.

34 Scutchfield SB: All-terrain vehicles: injuries and prevention. Clin Orthop Relat Res 2003;61–72.

35 Mueller FO, Blyth CS: Fatalities from head and cervical spine injuries occurring in tackle football: 40 years' experience. Clin Sports Med 1987;6:185–196.

36 Meeuwisse W, Bahr R: A systematic approach to sports injury prevention; in Bahr R, Engebretsen L (eds): Sports Injury Prevention: Handbook of Sports Medicine. Oxford, Wiley-Blackwell, 2009, pp 7–16.

37 Schiff M, Caine D, O'Halleron R: Injury prevention in sports. Am J Lifestyle Med 2010;4:42–64

38 Lysens R, Steverlynck A, van den Auweele W, et al: The predictability of sports injuries. Sports Med 1984;1:6–10.

39 Meeuwisse W: Assessing causation in sport injury: a multifactorial model. Clin J Sport Med 1994;4:166–170.

40 Bahr R, Holme I: Risk factors for sports injuries – a methodological approach. Br J Sports Med 2003;37: 384–392.

41 Meeuwisse W, Tyreman H, Hagel B, Emery C: A dynamic model of etiology of sport injury: the recursive nature of risk and causation. Clin J Sports Med 2007;17:215–219.

42 Meeuwisse W, Hagel B: The multi-causality of injury – current concepts; in Verhagen E, van Mechelen W (eds): Sports Injury Research. London, Oxford University Press, 2010, pp 99–107.

43 Bahr R, Krosshaug T: Understanding injury mechanisms: a key component of preventing injuries in sport. Br J Sports Med 2005;39:324–329.

44 Caine D, Harmer P, Schiff M (eds): Epidemiology of Injury in Olympic Sports. Oxford, Wiley/Blackwell in association with the International Olympic Committee, 2009.

45 Wedderkopp N, Kaltoft M, Lundgaard B, Rosendahl M, Froberg K: Prevention of injuries in young female players in European team handball: a prospective intervention study. Scand J Med Sci Sports 1999;9:41–47.

46 Wedderkopp N, Kaltoft M, Holm R, Froberg K: Comparison of two intervention programmes in young female players in European handball – with and without ankle disc. Scand J Med Sci Sports 2003;13:371–375.

47 Verhagen E, van der Beek A, Twisk J, Bouter L, Bahr R, van Mechelen W: The effect of a proprioceptive balance board training program for the prevention of ankle sprains: a prospective controlled trial. Am J Sports Med 2004;32:1385–1393.

48 Emery CA, Cassidy JD, Klassen TP, Rosychuk RJ, Rowe BH: Effectiveness of a home-based balance-training program in reducing sports-related injuries among healthy adolescents: a cluster randomized controlled trial. Can Med Assoc J 2005;172:749–754.

49 McGuine TA, Keene JS: The effect of a balance training program on the risk of ankle sprains in high school athletes. Am J Sports Med 2006;34: 1103–1111.

50 Christy GR: Serious parasport injuries in Auckland, New Zealand. Emerg Med Australas 2005;17:163–166.

51 Taylor DM, Bennett D, Carter M, Garewal D, Finch C: Perceptions of surfboard riders regarding the need for protective headgear. Wilderness Environ Med 2005;16:75–80.

52 Committee on Injury and Poison Prevention; American Academy of Pediatrics. Skateboard and scooter injuries. Pediatrics 2002;109:542–543.

53 Bowman SM, Aitken ME, Helmkamp JC, Maham SA, Graham CJ: Impact of helmets on injuries to riders of all-terrain vehicles. Inj Prev 2009;15:3–7.

54 McCrory P, Meeuwisse W, Johnston K, Dvorak J, Aubry M, Molloy M, Cantu R: Consensus Statement on Concussion in Sport: the 3rd International Conference on Concussion in Sport held in Zurich, November 2008. Br J Sports Med 2009;43:i76–i84.

55 Finch C: A new framework for research leading to sports injury prevention. J Sci Med Sport 2006;9: 3–9.

Dennis J. Caine, PhD, Professor and Chairperson
Department of Physical Education, Exercise Science and Wellness
Hyslop Sports Center, Room 114B
2751 2nd Ave N, Stop 8235, Grand Forks, ND 58202-8235 (USA)
Tel. +1 701 777 4041, E-Mail dennis.caine@email.und.edu

Heggie TW, Caine DJ (eds): Epidemiology of Injury in Adventure and Extreme Sports.
Med Sport Sci. Basel, Karger, 2012, vol 58, pp 17–43

# The Epidemiology of Injury in Mountaineering, Rock and Ice Climbing

Volker Schöffl[a–d] · Audry Morrison[d] · Isabelle Schöffl[e] ·
Thomas Küpper[d, f]

[a]Department of Sport Orthopedics, Klinikum Bamberg, Bamberg, [b]Department of Trauma Surgery, Friedrich Alexander University, Erlangen-Nuremberg, Germany; [c]Medical Commission IFSC, Turin, Italy; [d]Medical Commission UIAA, Berne, Switzerland; [e]Department of Pediatrics, Klinikum Bamberg, Bamberg, and [f]Institute of Occupational and Social Medicine, Aachen Technical University, Aachen, Germany

**Abstract**

Climbing and mountaineering sports are gaining more and more public interest. This chapter reviews scientific studies on injuries and accidents in climbing and mountaineering sports to evaluate the danger of these sports and their specific injuries and preventive measures. An initial PubMed query was performed using the key words 'rock climbing', 'sport climbing', 'mountaineering', 'alpine injuries' and 'climbing injuries'. More than 500 extracted papers were analyzed which gave information on injury, mortality/fatality, prevention and risk factors. Cross-references were also scanned according to the above given criteria. Also the data sources of the UIAA and IFSC Medical Commissions were analyzed. Overall, alpine (traditional) climbing has a higher injury risk than sport climbing, especially indoor climbing. Alpine and ice climbing have more objective dangers which can affect climber safety. Overall injury rates are low, nevertheless fatalities do occur in all climbing disciplines. Altitude-related illnesses/injuries also occur in mountaineering. Most injuries in sport climbing are overstrain injuries of the upper extremity. In alpine climbing, injuries mostly occur through falls which affect the lower extremity. Objective reporting of the injury site and severity varied in most studies according to the injury definition and methodology used. This creates differences in the injury and fatality results and conclusions, which in turn makes inter-study comparisons difficult. In future studies, the UIAA MedCom score for mountain injuries should be used to guarantee inter-study comparability. Evidence in preventive measures is low and further studies must be performed in this field.



While mountaineering has a long tradition, rock climbing as a sport itself originated from it in the mid-1980s. Its popularity spread globally and diversified to include new categories like ice climbing, bouldering, speed and aid climbing. The style in which way a route is climbed (e.g. free or aid) and the difficulty of the route itself became more important than just to reach the summit. In mountaineering the routes to reach the summit became more and more difficult and extreme. With the increasing number of sport climbers the urge for competition climbing was born. In 1991 only a few countries participated in the first world championships, but by 2005 some 500 athletes from 55 countries competed. Two international bodies represent climbing and mountaineering: the UIAA (Union Internationale des Associations d'Alpinisme – International Mountaineering and Climbing Federation) and the IFSC (International Federation of Sport Climbing). While the UIAA is in charge of outdoor climbing and mountaineering concerns, as well as ski mountaineering and ice-climbing competitions, the IFSC looks after competition rock climbing and currently seeks recognition as an Olympic sport [1].

Rock-climbing sports at a high recreational level or elite level are known to place extreme forces on the distal extremities, especially the upper body [2]. Before 1986, published studies on rock-climbing injuries consisted of trauma reports sustained in falls (i.e. from 'trad' or 'big wall' >1,000 m climbs in Yosemite National Park, USA), or studies on the effects of altitude [3, 4]. However, from the late 1980s, researchers focused on the increasing number of overuse injuries to the hand and upper bodies of the new generation of dedicated rock climbers [3, 5–11]. During the past 10 years, several prospective rock-climbing studies have begun to examine sport-specific injuries and fatalities [12–14].

Mountaineering involves a wide range of activities, from hiking up to climbing peaks above 8,000 m. All these activities present different physiological demands and risks depending on climbing style, altitude, environmental conditions, climbing experience and more [4, 15–20]. Most studies on mountaineering fatalities and accidents report the fatality/accident rates per 1,000 climbers or per 1,000 summits, which are difficult to compare to the denominator 1,000 h of sports performance used in other disciplines. In this review we tried to adjust these numbers for comparison purposes.

For higher altitude not only the accident and fatality rate are important but the prevalence of altitude illness, which is between 28 and 34% above 4,000 m [21]. These illnesses can be a contributing factor to an injury, accident or death. They are characterized by shifts of internal body fluid being in places they should not be on exposure to altitude (i.e. brain, lungs). At 'high altitude' (5,000+ m), there is a risk that these altitude-induced internal fluid shifts may accumulate in the brain (high altitude cerebral edema – HACE), and/or in the lungs (high altitude pulmonary edema – HAPE). Both HAPE and HACE are potentially fatal.

As most climbers regularly participate in a number of climbing styles, and in recent times may train on indoor climbing walls and finger or campus boards, prospective injury studies in a single climbing style other than mountaineering are rare [5]. In general, there are five major types of climbing: (1) mountaineering (climbing on snow, rock or ice to reach a peak or summit, usually at moderate or high altitudes in remote areas); (2) traditional (alpine) rock climbing (which generally involves minimal exposure to rock or ice and usually occurs at relatively low or moderate elevations); (3) sport climbing (climbing on pre-equipped routes with little physical hazards, also including bouldering (ropeless climbing on boulders of up to 8 m height)); (4) indoor climbing (including competition climbing), and (5) vertical ice climbing (including frozen waterfalls).

The borders in between these disciplines are fluctuant and many climbers regularly participate in more than one climbing subdiscipline. As many studies analyze traditional and sport climbing together, these two will be discussed in one group together in the further analysis.

Our search procedures included an initial PubMed query using the key words 'rock climbing', 'sport climbing', 'mountaineering', 'alpine injuries' and 'climbing injuries'. More than 500 extracted papers were analyzed which gave information on injury, mortality, prevention and risk factors. Cross-references were also scanned according to the above given criteria. The data sources of the UIAA and IFSC Medical Commissions were also analyzed.

### Who Is Affected by Injury?

*Traditional and Sport Climbing*

In general the studies show an inhomogeneous gender distribution of injury rate (table 1). Jones et al. [7] found an odds ratio of 1.01 of male gender for a rock-climbing injury, whereas Josephsen et al. [14] found little or no influence of gender (table 1). Neuhof et al. [22] found that more male climbers than female climbers had a history of at least one climbing injury during the observed period ($p = 0.50$). Nelson et al. [23] report a mean age for rock-climbing injuries of 26 years (95% CI 24.89–27.11) and Schöffl et al. [24] of 28.3 years (95% CI 13–52).

Analyzing injury frequency, Backe et al. [25] report 4.2 injuries/1,000 climbing hours, overuse injuries accounting for 93% of all injuries. Neuhof et al. [22] excluded overuse injuries and found an injury rate of 0.2/1,000 h in 1,962 climbers. In another study, the mean number of injuries per climber was 2.3 (±0.14) and 17.9% reported no injuries [8]. Older studies (1988) report an injury risk of 0.2–0.4% per rock-climbing day in the Yosemite National Park, equaling 37.5 injuries/1,000 h of exposure [4].

*Indoor Climbing*

During the Climbing World Championships 2005, all significant injuries ($n = 4$) involved women [12] (table 2). A lower overall injury risk was observed for indoor climbing than for outdoor rock climbing. Limb [26] reported 0.027 injuries/1,000 h and Schöffl and Winkelmann [13] 0.079 injuries/1,000 h of performance. For indoor competition climbing an injury risk of 3.1/1,000 h is reported [12].

**Table 1.** Injuries and fatalities in traditional and sport climbing. Modified from Schöffl et al. [5]

| Study | Type of climbing/ geographical location | Study design n | Cause of injury/location |
|---|---|---|---|
| Bowie et al. [4] | Traditional climbing, bouldering; Yosemite Valley, USA (some rock walls 1,000 m high) | Data collection in the ER of the central hospital within the area n = 220, I, R | Mainly lead climbing falls, mostly lower extremity |
| Addiss and Baker [15] | Mountaineering and traditional climbing; US national parks (includes snow and ice terrain) | Rock-climbing injuries that were reported to US national park services (1981–82) n =127, R | 75% falls |
| Schussmann et al. [32] | Mountaineering and traditional climbing (Grand Tetons, Wyo., USA) | Data collection through national park registration from 1981 to 1986; representing 43,631 climbers, 108 accidents, all mountaineering activities n = 108, R | More mountaineering accidents than rock climbing |
| Rooks et al. [39] | Recreational rock climbers, Ga., USA | 39 recreational climbers n = 39, Q, R | Mostly upper extremity, 6 climbers climbing beyond the sport level sustained a major injury from a fall, 35 sustained at least one significant injury |
| Paige et al. [19] | Traditional climbing, sport climbing | n = 94, R, Q, I including overstrain injuries | Mainly lead climbing, falling when alpine climbing, injuries from hard moves in sport climbing; upper extremity, fingers especially affected |
| Rohrbourgh et al. [3] | Competition rock climbers at US national championships | n = 42 elite rock climbers, only overuse syndromes R, Q, E | Injuries mostly in upper limbs |
| Schöffl et al. [34] | European climbers | n = 604 (injured climbers) I, E, P (4 years) | Upper extremity 67% |
| Logan et al. [10] | Rock climbers, UK | n = 545, Q, R members of the Climbers Club of Great Britain, examined prevalence of hand injuries | |
| Gerdes et al. [8] | Rock climbing | n = 1,887, Q, R 2,472 injuries, including overuse injuries | Upper extremity 57.6% |

| Injuries/1,000 h sport performance | Injury severity (NACA score) | Fatality | Risk evaluation |
|---|---|---|---|
| 37.5[a] | Majority of minor severity using ISS score; 95% ISS <13; 5% ISS 13–75 | 13 of 220 subjects had severe injuries, of which 11 were fatal (5.9%); case fatality rate 6% | Bias of injuries presented may reflect more serious injuries requiring ER treatment |
| NS | 28% NACA seven (fatal)[b] | 36 (28%); injuries on snow and ice were more likely to be fatal | Potentially high-risk activity |
| 0.56 for injuries; 0.13 for fatalities; incidence 2.5 accidents/1,000 mountaineers/year or 5.6 injuries/10,000 h of mountaineering | 23% of the injuries were fatal (NACA 7)[b] | 25 fatal, 23% case fatality rate; fatality rate 0.13/1,000 h | Mountaineering was of a higher risk than rock climbing; climbing education and experience were considered preventative factors in accidents and injuries |
| NS | NS | 6 (15%) had a major injury from a fall | NS |
| NS | NS | None as retrospective questionnaire | No major difference between alpine and sport climbing |
| NS | NS | None | No significant relationship between overuse injuries and years of climbing or difficulty level |
| NS | Mostly NACA 1–2, only 0.8% severe injuries (NACA 4 or 5) | None | Severe injuries were rare |
| NS | Mostly NACA 1 and 2[b] | None reported as it was a retrospective survey on hand injuries | Climbing score higher in injury group (including overstrains) ($p < 0.05$) |
| NS | 20% no injury; 60% NACA 1; 20% >NACA 1[b] | None reported as it was a retrospective survey | Traditional ($p < 0.01$) and solo climbing ($p < 0.01$) had more injuries. Injuries even distributed between indoors and outdoors |

**Table 1.** Continued

| Study | Type of climbing/ geographical location | Study design n | Cause of injury/location |
|---|---|---|---|
| Smith [89] | Review on alpine-climbing injuries | Review | Falls are the most frequent injury cause |
| German Alpine Club [69] | All climbing disciplines | n = 1,491, R Reports on all climbing accidents reported to the DAV insurance cover (2004–05) | |
| Josephsen et al. [14] | Bouldering (indoor and outdoor) Calif., USA | n = 152, P, Q cross-sectional cohort study | |
| Jones et al. [7] | Rock climbers (indoor and outdoor) | n = 201, R, Q cross-sectional study | 10% acute through falls, 33% overuse injuries 28% acute through strenuous move |
| Nelson and McKenzie [23] | Rock-climbing injuries (indoor and outdoor) | n = 846, R 846 cases being treated at US NEISS hospitals were collected and 40,282 injuries for the USA estimated (1990–2007) | Lower extremity mostly affected |
| Backe et al. [25] | All climbing disciplines | n = 355, R, Q 1.5-year period (2005/2006) | 93% overuse injuries, 7% traumatic, overall mostly upper limb, 50% of traumatic lower limb |
| Neuhof et al. [44] | Sport climbing | n = 1,962, R, Q reviewed 5 years of sport climbing injuries | Upper (42.6%) and lower (41.3%) limbs equally effected (699 injuries) |

DAV = German Alpine Club; ER = emergency room; ISS = Injury Severity Score; NACA = National Advisory Committee for Aeronautics; NEISS = National Electronic Injury Surveillance System, I = interview, P = prospective, Q = questionnaire, R = retrospective, E = physical examination.

[a] Injuries/fatalities per 1,000 h calculated by the authors according to the information given in the study.

[b] NACA score graded by the authors according to the information given in the study.

| Injuries/1,000 h sport performance | Injury severity (NACA score) | Fatality | Risk evaluation |
|---|---|---|---|
| NS | NS | NS | Falling injuries are more severe in alpine climbing |
| NS | NS | NS | 12% of all accidents in mountain sports are from rock and ice climbing: 48% of these from alpine climbing, 29% sport climbing, 9% indoor climbing, 6% ice climbing, 1% bouldering |
| NS | NS | None | Few differences between injuries experienced between indoor and outdoor |
| NS | NS | None reported as it was a retrospective study | Climbing frequency and difficulty are associated with incidence of overuse injuries |
| Measures of participation and frequency of exposure to rock climbing are not given | Mostly NACA 1–2[b], 11.3% hospitalization | None reported as it was a retrospective study | Overexertion injuries more likely on the upper body |
| 4.2 (including overuse injuries)<br>0.29 for acute injuries | NS | None reported as it was a retrospective study | Overweight and bouldering implies increased injury risk |
| 0.2 | NACA1 36.1%<br>NACA2 38.3%<br>NACA3 24.6%<br>NACA4/5 1%<br>NACA 6/7 0<br>UIAA1 0 (excluded)<br>UIAA2 81.4%<br>UIAA3 18.2%<br>UIAA4/6 0.4% | None reported as it was a retrospective study | Years of climbing experience ($p < 0.01$), difficulty level ($p < 0.01$) and climbing time per week ($p < 0.01$) correlated with injury rate |

**Table 2.** Injuries and fatalities in indoor and competition climbing. Modified from Schöffl et al. [5]

| Study | Type of climbing/ location | Study design n | Cause of injury/location |
|---|---|---|---|
| Limb [26] | 90 indoor climbing walls in England, Wales and Scotland | n = 55, significant injuries reported with 1.021 million visits R, Q | Mostly upper limb |
| Schöffl and Winkelmann [13] | Indoor climbing walls, Germany | n = 25,163 registrants to indoor climbing walls P, Q | |
| Wright et al. [11] | Overuse injuries in indoor climbing at World Championships Birmingham, UK, 1999 | n = 295, R, Q spectators and competitors | 44% had overuse injuries, mostly fingers |
| Schöffl and Küpper [12] | Indoor competition climbing, World Championships, Germany, 2005 | n = 443 climbers (273 M; 170 F) from 55 countries P, E | 18 acute injuries of which 4 were significant |
| Josephsen et al. [14] | Bouldering (indoor and outdoor), Calif., USA | n = 152, P, Q cross-sectional cohort study | Overuse |
| German Alpine Club [69] | All climbing disciplines | n = 1,491, R. Reports on all climbing accidents reported to the DAV insurance cover (2004–05) | |
| Jones et al. [7] | Rock climbers (indoors and outdoors) | n = 201, R, Q cross-sectional study | 10% acute through falls; 33% overuse injuries; 28% acute through strenuous move |

DAV = German Alpine Club; F = females; M = males; NACA = National Advisory Committee for Aeronautics, I = interview, P = prospective, Q = questionnaire, R = retrospective, E = physical examination.
[a] Injuries/fatalities per 1,000 h calculated by the authors according to the information given in the study.
[b] NACA score graded by the authors according to the information given in the study.

| Injuries/1,000 h sport performance | Injury severity (NACA score) | Fatality | Risk evaluation |
|---|---|---|---|
| 0.027[a] | All >NACA 1[a]; none NACA 7 | None | Climbing walls with very low injury rate; injury rate not related to any identified wall design or safety feature |
| 0.079[a] | 3 NACA 2; 1 NACA 3 | None | Indoor climbing is a very low risk sport for acute injuries |
| NS | NACA 1–2[b] | None | Climbing harder routes correlated to overuse injuries ($p < 0.01$) |
| 3.1 | 16 NACA 1; 1 NACA 2; 1 NACA 3 | None | Indoor rock climbing has a low injury risk and a good safety profile |
| NS | NS | None | Few differences between indoor and outdoor |
| NS | NS | NS | 12% of all accidents in mountain sports are from rock and ice climbing: 48% of theses alpine climbing, 29% sport climbing, 9% indoor climbing, 6% ice climbing, 1% bouldering |
| NS | NS | None | Climbing frequency and difficulty are associated with incidence of overuse injuries |

**Table 3.** Injuries and fatalities in ice climbing. Modified from Schöffl et al. [5]

| Study | Type of climbing/ location | Study design n | Cause of injury/location |
|---|---|---|---|
| Mosimann [64] | Ice climbing, Switzerland | n = 46, R<br>Outcome of ice climbers rescued by Swiss mountain rescue service over 6 years | Most frequent injury causes were falls (55%), but no fatal injuries were sustained through falls |
| Schöffl et al. [27] | Ice climbing, international | n = 88, R, Q<br>3 years | 95 injuries, overuse syndromes |
| American Alpine Club [16] | All climbing accidents, USA | n = 11,089,R,<br>Alpine club records from 1951 to 2003 reported 6,111 accidents (5,931 unharmed) | |
| German Alpine Club [69] | All climbing disciplines | n = 1491, R<br>Reports on all climbing accidents reported to the DAV insurance cover (2004–05) | |
| Canadian Alpine Club [17] | All climbing accidents, Canada | n = 2,003 R<br>Alpine club records from 1951 to 2003 reported 958 accidents<br>715 injured, 163 occurred on ice | |

DAV = German Alpine Club; NACA = National Advisory Committee for Aeronautics, I = interview, P = prospective, Q = questionnaire, R = retrospective, E = physical examination.
[a] NACA score graded by the authors according to the information given in the study.

*Ice Climbing*

In ice climbing [27], female climbers were injured more often (76.9%) than males (58.7%) (table 3). Schöffl et al. [27] report an injury risk of 4.07/1,000 h of performance.

*Mountaineering*

McIntosh et al. [28] found little or no influence of gender on risk of injury (table 4). Recreational injuries in Washington State Park were mostly in males [29]. Typically, two age groups are involved in mountaineering accidents: climbers from 20 to 35 years suffering from trauma and climbers from 45 to 55 years who in addition also have a relevant number of non-traumatic problems [30, 31]. In fatal accidents, significantly more men are involved than women ($p < 0.05$) [30].

Schussmann et al. [32] reported an incidence of 2.5 accidents/1,000 mountaineers and year or 0.56/1,000 h of mountaineering. Most studies on mountaineering fatalities and accidents present the injury/fatality number per 1,000 climbers or per 1,000

| Injuries/1,000 h sport performance | Injury severity (NACA score) | Fatality | Risk evaluation |
|---|---|---|---|
| | 31% NACA 0; 42% NACA 2–3; 8% NACA 4; 6%NACA 5; 13% NACA 7 | Case fatality rate 13% | Fatality rate in ice climbing is higher than in mountaineering and rock climbing |
| 4.07 for NACA 1–3 | 2.87/1,000 h NACA 1; 1.2/1,000 h NACA 2/3; none >NACA 3 | None reported as retrospective study | Ice climbing is not a sport with a high risk of injury; 61% injuries occurred while leading, 24% following |
| NS | 53% NACA 0[a]; 12% NACA 7[a]; 4% NACA[a] accidents on ice | 1,373 fatal accidents overall | |
| NS | NS | NS | 12% of all accidents in mountain sports are from rock and ice climbing: 48% of theses alpine climbing; 29% sport climbing; 9% indoor climbing; 6% ice climbing; 1% bouldering |
| NS | NS | 292 fatal injuries, 30 fatal ice-climbing injuries occurred over a 30-year period | |

summits, making comparison with studies reporting injuries 1,000 h of sports performance difficult (table 4).

## Where Does Injury Occur?

*Anatomical Location*

Traditional and Sport Climbing

Unfortunately, many scientific climbing papers present case studies or common hand injuries [9, 24, 33–38] and are therefore not suitable for injury distribution analysis. So far, most research indicates that the upper extremity to be the most injured body regions in non-alpine rock climbing [8, 19, 22, 24, 25, 27, 39, 40]. Schöffl et al. [35] analyzed 604 injured climbers (sport climbing, indoor climbing) and reported 247 of 604 (40.9%) injuries involved the hand (table 5). Two studies that analyzed climbing injuries treated in American hospitals or emergency rooms [4,

**Table 4.** Injuries and fatalities in Mountaineering. Modified from Schöffl et al. [5]

| Study | Type of climbing/location (includes snow and ice terrain) | Study design n | Cause of injury/location |
|---|---|---|---|
| Addiss and Baker [15] | Mountaineering and traditional climbing, US national parks | rock-climbing injuries that were reported to US national park services (1981–82) n=127, R | 75% falls |
| Schussmann et al. [32] | Mountaineering and traditional climbing, Grand Tetons, Wyo., USA | Data collection through national park registration, n=108, R | More mountaineering accidents than rock climbing |
| Malcom [74] | Mountaineering, Mount Cook, New Zealand | n = 33, R Fatality analysis on Mount Cook | |
| Stephens et al. [29] | Washington State Park, USA | n = 535, R case incidence reports, recreational injuries | |
| Monasterio [70] | Mountaineering and alpine rock climbing in New Zealand, maximum altitude 4,000 m | n = 44, P, Q injuries over 4 years among mountaineers (40 M, 4 F) | |
| Firth et al. [75] | Mountaineers, Sherpas and climbers attempting to climb Mount Everest, 8850 m, highest point in the world | n = 28,276, R Search of Himalayan database and other records from 1921 to 2006; analysis of mortality among n = 28,276 where 192 deaths occurred | n = 113 died from objective falls or hazards; n = 52 non-traumatic (sudden death, altitude illness, hypothermia); n = 27 body never found |
| German Alpine Club [69] | All climbing disciplines that were covered by the insurance provider for the German Alpine Club | n = 1,491, R Reports on all climbing accidents reported to the DAV insurance cover (2004–05) | |
| American Alpine Club [16] | All climbing accidents, USA | n = 11,089, R Alpine club records from 1951 to 2003 reported 6,111 accidents (5,931 unharmed) | |
| Canadian Alpine Club [17] | All climbing accidents, Canada | n = 2,003, R Alpine club records from 1951 to 2003 reported 958 accidents 715 injured, 163 occurred on ice | |

| Injuries/1,000 h sport performance | Injury severity (NACA score) | Fatality | Risk evaluation |
|---|---|---|---|
| NS | 28% NACA 7 (fatal)[a] | 36 (28%) injuries on snow and ice were more likely to be fatal | Mountaineering was potentially a high-risk activity compared with rock climbing |
| 0.56 for injuries; 0.13 for fatalities | 23% of the injuries were fatal (NACA 7)[b] | 25 fatal case fatality rate: 23% | Author concluded mountaineering of higher risk than pure rock climbing |
| NS | NS | 0.12 for fatalities[a] or 1.87/1,000 exposure days | Mountaineering was associated with a high risk compared with other activities |
| NS | NS | Hiking was the most common activity during time of death 58%, 26% in mountaineering | |
| NS | NS | 5 NACA 7 (fatal) [8.7%]; 1 death was unrelated to climbing, 2 fell into crevasses, 2 died by climbing misadventure (1 climber was climbing alone) | Mountain climbing was associated with a high risk of serious injury and mortality; baseline climbing experience was 5–7 years |
| NS | NS | Mountaineers had a mortality rate of 1.3% | Debilitating symptoms of high altitude pulmonary edema associated with descent from summit; subsequent deaths associated with late arrival at summit and fatigue |
| NS | NS | NS | 12% of all accidents occurred in mountain sports are from rock climbing: 48% of these alpine climbing; 29% sport climbing; 9% indoor climbing; 1% bouldering |
| NS | 53% NACA 0[b]; 12% NACA 7[b]; 4% NACA[b] accidents on ice | 1,373 fatal accidents | |
| NS | NS | 292 fatal injuries; 30 fatal ice-climbing injuries occurred over a 30-year period | |

**Table 4.** Continued

| Study | Type of climbing/location (includes snow and ice terrain) | Study design n | Cause of injury/location |
|---|---|---|---|
| Hearns et al. [90] | Mountaineers who were patients at a specialist spinal hospital in Scotland | n = 21, R, Q 21 from 1,400 patients identified with spinal injuries from mountaineering over 10 years | 4 rock climbing, 6 winter climbing, 1 other |
| McIntosh et al. [28] | School teaching outdoor training and wilderness skills taught at the National Outdoor Leadership School, Lander, Wyo., USA | n = 996 medical incidents R, 2002–05 | |
| McIntosh et al. [71] | Mountaineering Mount McKinley (or Mount Denali) in Alaska, 6,194 m | n = 96, R fatalities from 1903 to 2006 | |
| McLennan and Ungersma [41] | Mountaineering in Sierra Nevada, Columbia; peaks up to 5,700 m | n = 215 mountaineering accidents R, 5 years of accidents and their possible causes when climbing class V routes | 94 involved ankle and lower tibia, 17 deaths mostly involved head injuries |
| Küpper [30] | European Alps (Switzerland, Austria) | R, n = 2,730 helicopter rescue operations, 4,139 diagnoses | 72.8% trauma (falls and collisions)/27.2% non-traumatic (0.5% alcohol; 0.2% suicide); of trauma diagnoses: 31.8% head/vertebral column, 12.5% trunk, 18.9% upper extremities, 28.5% legs |

DAV = German Alpine Club; F = females; M = males; NACA = National Advisory Committee for Aeronautics, I = interview, P = prospective, Q = questionnaire, R = retrospective, E = physical examination.
[a] Injuries/fatalities per 1,000 h calculated by the authors according to the information given in the study.
[b] NACA score graded by the authors according to the information given in the study.

32] reported that most climbing injuries involved the lower extremities and resulted from big swings into the wall or big falls [4, 23]. The authors suggest that these findings may be partially explained by the minor nature of many rock climbing-related injuries recalled by participants in the other surveys. In another recent study on rock-climbing injuries, traumatic injuries involved the lower extremities (foot, toe and ankle) in 50%, while upper extremities accounted for 36% of the injuries [25].

| Injuries/1,000 h sport performance | Injury severity (NACA score) | Fatality | Risk evaluation |
|---|---|---|---|
| NS | NS | None, as study was of survivors with spinal injuries from mountaineering | Incidence of spinal cord injury less than in overall group of spinal injury patients<br>Most of the 21 subjects studied had other significant and potentially distracting injuries |
| 0.071 NACA 1[a]; 0.074 NACA 1–3[a]; 0.0056% NACA 2–3[a] | 92% NACA 1[b]; 7.6% NACA 2–3[b]; none >NACA 3[b] | None | |
| 0.063 for fatalities[a] | NS | 3.08/1,000 summit attempts, or 100/1 million exposure days on Mount Denali | Fatality rate is declining |
| NS | NS | 17 deaths, mostly from head injuries | Poor acclimatization with acute mountain sickness and hypothermia found in 104 patients, resulting in judgmental errors |
| NS | 17.3% NACA I–II, 43.6% NACA III, NACA IV–VI 27.4%, 5.2% NACA VII (Western > Eastern Alps) | 142 (5.2%) injuries and non-traumatic incidences were fatal | Significant differences of the risk between different alpine disciplines (not exactly defined since the total number of climbers or hours of climbing is unknown) |

Neuhof et al. [22] found an even injury distribution between the upper (42.6%) and lower extremities (41.3%) (table 1).

## Indoor Climbing

Limb [26] as well as Wright et al. [11] report mostly about upper limb injuries for indoor climbing (table 2).

**Table 5.** The 10 most frequent locations of injuries in sport and indoor climbing (n = 604), 1/1998–2/2001

| | |
|---|---|
| Fingers | 247 (41.0%) |
| Elbow/forearm | 81 (13.4%) |
| Foot | 55 (9.1%) |
| Hand | 47 (7.8%) |
| Spine/trunk | 43 (7.1%) |
| Skin | 42 (6.9%) |
| Shoulder | 30 (5.0%) |
| Knee | 22 (3.6%) |
| Other | 37 (6.1%) |
| Polytrauma | 5 (0.8%) |

Ice Climbing

The most injured body regions in ice climbing are the head and the upper extremities [27] (table 6).

Mountaineering

In a recent study, which included 2,730 alpine rescue operations, 72.8% of diagnoses were trauma and 16.6% concerning internal medicine or neurology [30]. Almost 36% of the trauma diagnoses involved the head or vertebral column, 14.3% trunk, 25.5% legs, and 14.1% arms. In 1.8%, a polytrauma was present. Almost half (45.2%) of the internal/neurological diagnoses affected the cardiovascular system [30] (table 4). In another study [41], 94 of 215 injuries involved the ankle and the lower tibia, the 17 deaths mostly involved head injuries.

*Environmental Location*

Climbing Sports

Designing scientific studies that account for all environmental injury variables related to outdoor climbing is difficult [42]. Injuries at indoor climbing walls have more controlled sport-specific variables and are better documented (table 2). More injuries are found in traditional and alpine climbing than in sport or indoor climbing [5, 8] (table 1). Gerdes et al. [8] report a similar distribution of indoor and outdoor climbing injuries, which is in contradiction to Schöffl et al. [5, 13]. Very few injuries occur during climbing competitions [8, 12] and indoor climbing (table 2).

Mountaineering

Küpper's study [30] provides the most detailed data on environmental location – at least for the European Alps. A little more than 26% of all accidents were located at NACA 3D terrain, which means that accessibility is limited and takes time [30]. 8.5% were in difficult access terrain while 5.9% were in very difficult or extreme terrain.

**Table 6.** Location of injury in ice climbing (n = 120)

| | |
|---|---|
| Head | 49 (40.8%) |
| Finger | 16 (13.3%) |
| Leg | 15 (12.5%) |
| Foot | 6 (5%) |
| Arm | 6 (5%) |
| Shoulder | 3 (2.5%) |
| Chest | 3 (2.5%) |
| Back | 2 (1.7%) |
| Neck | 1 (0.8%) |
| Perianal | 1 (0.8%) |
| Others | 18 (15%) |

There were significant differences between summer and winter climbing injury rates ($p < 0.05$) (table 4).

### When Does Injury Occur?

*Injury Onset*

A distinction between acute injuries and chronic injuries (overuse syndromes) is important. Nevertheless, this distinction may be difficult as some injuries, for example tenosynovitis in the fingers, may have an acute or chronic onset [6]. Most injuries in traditional climbing are acute and result from a fall [4, 15]. Sport and indoor climbing show an almost even distribution between acute injuries from performing a strenuous move and chronic injuries (table 2). Schöffl et al. [27] report similar findings for ice climbing, with most acute injuries presenting while lead climbing. In mountaineering the vast majority are acute injuries (table 3, 4).

*Chronometry*

Few studies provide data on the timing of injury. In Yosemite National Park more rock-climbing injuries occurred in spring (47%) than in summer or autumn [4]. Injuries were disproportionately higher on weekends and time of injury was distributed evenly with the highest frequency at noon [4]. Most injuries in recreational activities in Washington State Park occurred during the summer months between noon and 6.00 p.m. [29]. This finding is expected as more climbers climb in summer and during daylight than at nighttime in winter. In alpine climbing the peak of injuries or accidents is at noon or early afternoon with 70.1% of all injuries occurring between 11 a.m. and 5 p.m., and most of these between 1 and 3 p.m. [43]. Most authors interpret these data as reflecting decreasing mental and physical performance after hours of climbing.

**Table 7.** The most frequent injuries and overuse syndromes in sport climbers (n=604), 1998–2002

| | |
|---|---|
| Pulley injury | 122 |
| Tenosynovitis | 42 |
| Epicondylitis | 51 |
| Joint capsular damage | 37 |
| •Skin laceration | 34 |
| Back problems | 24 |
| Knee problems | 14 |
| Others | 281 |

## What Is the Outcome?

*Injury Type*

Traditional, Sport Climbing and Indoor Climbing

Most authors [8, 23, 25, 35, 44] report that fractures, strains and sprains are predominant. Chronic overuse injuries occur most often on the upper extremities at the elbow and the fingers [8, 22, 35]. As hand and finger injuries are the most common (table 7), many studies focus on these [9, 24, 33–38, 45]. Schöffl et al. [35] found as the most common climbing injury the closed pulley rupture and the most common overuse injuries were epicondylitis and tenosynovitis of the finger flexor tendons. These pulley injuries are almost rock climbing-specific pathologies and have been studied extensively [24, 46–48]. Other finger injuries which are climbing-specific include 'lumbrical shift syndrome' [49], 'extensor hood syndrome' [50], 'epiphyseal fractures' [51], 'flap irritation phenomenon (FLIP) syndrome' [52], 'finger amputations – rope-tangling injuries' [36], morbus Dupuytren [53] and acute problems because of osteoarthritis of the fingers [38, 54, 55]. In recent publications, back problems ('climbers back' [56]), shoulder pathologies (SLAP and biceps tendon tears [57–59]) as well as feet deformations are evolving [60–62].

Ice Climbing

Most acute injuries in ice climbing are open wounds (55.2%) and hematomas (21.9%) [27] (table 8).

Mountaineering

Mountaineering tends to be associated with higher graded trauma, multiple fractures, severe wounds and polytraumatic patients (table 4). Küpper [30] analyzed 2,730 rescue operations. The 72.8% of trauma cases showed a significantly higher severity than those in sports climbing, especially more fractures, severe wounds, and polytraumatic patients. Due to high altitude there were diagnoses which do not occur in other

**Table 8.** Ice-climbing injuries (n = 102)

| | |
|---|---|
| Open wounds | 53 (52%) |
| Haematoma | 21 (20.6%) |
| Frostbite | 9 (8.8%) |
| Fractures | 2 (1.9%) |
| Other | 17 (16.7%) |

climbing sports, e.g. altitude disease (2.5%) or 'alpine' diagnoses like hypothermia, exhaustion, or heat stroke [30].

*Injury Severity*

Traditional and Sport Climbing

As shown in table 1, most injuries in climbing studies were of minor severity, although the scores and definitions employed were inconsistent. A post-hoc NACA classification of the injuries reported in these studies was reported by Schöffl et al. [63] (table 1). Overall, the majority of injuries in outdoor and alpine climbing were of minor severity (NACA 1–2).

Indoor Climbing

Two large-scale studies [13, 26] analyzed indoor-climbing injuries. Limb's [26] survey reported 55 accidents, from 1.02 million climbing wall visits, and no fatalities. Schöffl and Winkelmann [13] prospectively surveyed 25,163 registrants at ten climbing walls. Only four significant injuries (NACA 3, UIAA 2) were found and no fatalities (table 2).

Ice Climbing

For ice climbing, few data on injuries and accidents exist. Schöffl et al. [27] found mainly NACA 1 injuries, and no injury score above NACA 3. Of 46 ice climbers rescued over 6 years, Mosimann [64] found 31% had no injury (NACA 0), 42% had NACA 2–3 injuries, 8% had NACA 4, 6% NACA 5, and 13% (6 climbers) had a fatal injury (NACA 7) (table 3).

Mountaineering

Few mountaineering studies provide exact injury scores. Küpper [30] reported 43.6% of all accidents classified as NACA 3 and only 17.3% as NACA 0–2, but 27.4% as NACA 4–6. 5.2% were NACA 7 (= dead).

*Clinical Outcome – Catastrophic Injuries (Fatalities)*

Traditional and Sport Climbing

Recent statistics of the German Alpine Club (DAV) reported 7 deaths during 2006 and 2007 [65]. These statistics do not differentiate between traditional, ice and sport climbing. A retrospectively conducted study on mountaineering reported an incidence of 0.13 fatalities/1,000 h [32]. For alpine climbing, Bowie et al. [4] documented that 13 of 220 injured climbers died – a case fatality rate of 6%. This case fatality rate was much smaller than older American records from 1951 to 1960 that recorded 41% [66], 23% for the Grand Tetons [32] in 1982, and 8% for the Sierra Nevada [41]. Schussmann et al. [32] calculated, based on 25 fatalities in his study, a fatality rate of 0.13/1,000 h or a case fatality rate of 23%. Bowie et al.'s [4] Yosemite results are in accordance with the results of Hubicka [67] for European climbing areas. The analyses in these climbing injury studies were conducted retrospectively using questionnaires, and therefore may be prone to recall bias. The 'older' studies (20 years ago) [4, 15, 32] reported the most severe injuries and highest fatality rates, while recently a prospectively conducted study on bouldering [14] reported no fatalities at all (table 1).

### Ice Climbing

The Canadian Alpine Club [68] and the American Alpine Club [16] have statistically recorded and analyzed all mountain accidents since 1951. In the USA, up to the year 2005, there were 6,111 incidents involving 11,089 mountaineers recorded by the American Alpine Club [16]. Of these were 1,373 (12%) fatalities (NACA 7). 254 (4%) accidents happened in ice, though no further evaluation of the ice-climbing injuries was provided. As 4% of all injuries are associated with ice climbing, also 4% of all fatalities can be assumed to be ice climbing-related. This would calculate to 55 fatally ice-climbing injuries in 54 years, or 1 ice-climbing fatality per year within the USA. During the same time frame, 958 accidents in 2,003 mountaineers were recorded in Canada [68]. 715 (36%) mountaineers were injured, 292 (15%) fatal. 163 (17%) of the Canadian accidents occurred on 'ice' terrain. In 30 years, 92 mountaineers were injured while ice climbing, 30 fatally. The German Alpine Club (DAV) records ice-climbing accidents that are reported to their insurance carrier. In the years 2004–2005, 150 climbing accidents were recorded, 12% of all accidents in mountain sports (1,270) [69]. Alpine mixed climbing accounted for 8% of all accidents and water ice climbing for 6%. It is not possible to precisely determine the death risk from these numbers, as the absolute number of ice climbers in these areas is unknown. The major ice-climbing countries, Switzerland and Canada, report about 1 death per year [64, 68].

### Mountaineering

Monasterio [70] prospectively surveyed 46 rock climbers/mountaineers over 4 years to determine the type and frequency of accidents. He reported 5 deaths – 1 unrelated to climbing, 2 in avalanche, and 2 from climbing 'misadventure'. Küpper [30] found significantly more fatal accidents in men than women ($p < 0.05$), which may be a consequence of a higher risk acceptance in men. McIntosh et al. [71] reviewed mountaineering fatalities on Mount McKinley, Alaska (6,194 m). In recent years the fatality rate has declined to 3.08/1,000 summit attempts. They found this fatality rate 20 times higher than those given for trekkers hiking in Nepal [72] and even higher than those for English and Welsh mountaineers [73]. McIntosh et al. [71] adjusted denominators to allow comparison and reported a fatality rate of 100/1 million exposure days on Mount McKinley, or a fatality rate of 0.063/1,000 h. Malcom [74] reported 1.87/1,000 days mountaineering fatalities on Mount Cook in New Zealand, or 0.12 fatalities/1,000 h of mountaineering. This figure seems extremely high and may be the product of estimated exposure days based on hut night stays, rather than actual climbing days [71].

Firth et al. [75] calculated a mortality rate of 1.3% when examining causes of mortality among those who climbed Mount Everest from 1921 to 2006 (192 died from 28,276). Pollard and Clarke [76] found that at extreme altitude, 70–80% of mountaineering deaths were related to environmental factors. Salisbury [77] and Salisbury and Hawley [78] identified mortality rates between 0 and 0.126 deaths for every 100 mountaineers climbing above 6,000 m. In recent years the mortality in mountaineering has declined [79]. On 8,000 m peaks, ascent success rates declined with summit height, but overall death rates, and death rates during descent from the summit, increased with summit height [75, 80].

*Economic Cost*

Traditional and Sport Climbing

Climbers often do not seek a doctor's advice but undergo self-therapy [1, 7]. Gerdes et al. [8] found that only one third of the climbers even sought medical treatment. Neuhof et al. [22] found in sport climbers that 29% of the injuries were followed by a period where the climbers were incapable to work for an average time of 27.7 ± 41.6 days (range 1–300). More than a tenth (11.7%) of injuries required inpatient admission with a mean duration of 11.1 ± 16.4 days (range 1–120). 14% of injuries resulted in permanent damage including functional deficits (n = 56), pain (n = 33), deformities (n = 12), skin scars (n = 9) and psychosis (n = 1). Bowie et al. [4] give exact numbers on cost of injury, although the numbers must be considered as being from over 20 years ago (1988). The average clinic medical expense from climbers was USD 233.

Ice Climbing

In one ice-climbing study [27], 27.3% of injuries required a doctor's attendance; only a few (5.7%) needed hospitalization. Permanent damage occurred in 22.7% of the injury cases.

## What Are the Risk Factors?

For injury-intervention and rehabilitation programs to be effective, an in-depth knowledge of injury risk factors is paramount.

*Intrinsic Factors*

Traditional and Sport Climbing

Few studies distinguish between male and female in risk willingness and risk management (table 1). Self-efficacy and sex differences (male higher) emerged as important predictors of risk in rock climbing in a psychological analysis [81], while it appears that experienced climbers are less motivated by sensation seeking or impulsivity. Neuhof et al. [22] found a higher injury rate (number of injuries divided by 1,000 h of sport participation) for female (0.23) than for male (0.19) climbers ($p = 0.83$). Age ($p = 0.63$) and body mass index ($p = 0.46$) had no influence on the development of an injury. Difficulty level ($p < 0.01$) and climbing experience ($p < 0.01$) were significant for the development of at least one climbing injury. Climbing experience ($r = 0.06$, $p < 0.01$) and difficulty level ($r = 0.08$, $p < 0.01$) also correlated with injury rate. In contrast, Josephsen et al. [14] found no relation of bouldering injuries to gender, years of climbing, body mass index or weight.

Ice Climbing

Body mass index correlated significantly ($p < 0.05$) with an increased risk of injury in ice climbing [27]. Overuse syndromes correlated significantly with ice-climbing level ($p < 0.01$) and the risk willingness while lead climbing on ice ($p < 0.01$). The younger (under 30 years) ice climbers had a higher injury incidence than did older climbers (over 50 years). More than 10 years of ice-climbing experience resulted in a lower injury risk.

Mountaineering

Küpper [30] found fatal accidents to be significantly greater in men than women ($p < 0.05$), which may be a consequence of a higher risk acceptance in men. There was a linear increase of non-traumatic emergencies with the patient's age ($p = 0.94$). Risk tolerance and preexisting diseases are important factors of the age-depending pattern of incidence in younger and older alpine climbers [30]. Climbers from Asia had the greatest odds of dying on Denali [71], while the death rate on Mount Everest is higher in climbers than in Sherpas [75].

*Extrinsic Factors*

Traditional and Sport Climbing

Jones et al. [7] found that the frequency of all forms of climbing behavior were associated with overuse injuries. Josephsen et al. [14] found in boulderers no relation of injuries to years of climbing and no correlation to injury incidence to the use of spotters, numbers of spotters, height of average boulder, height of tallest boulder climbed, use of pads or number of pads. Neuhof et al. [44] found that climbing time per week is significant ($p < 0.01$) for the development of at least one climbing injury and also correlates with the injury rate ($p < 0.01$).

Certain grip techniques in rock climbing are more prone for injuries than others. Schöffl et al. [47, 48] demonstrated on a cadaver model that the crimp grip is more prone to injure the A4 pulley, while eccentric movements injure the A2 pulley. Gerdes et al. [8] found that males were found to use helmets less ($p = 0.019$) than female climbers and use illicit substances more. The pattern of injury after rock-climbing falls is not determined by harness type [82]. Those climbers with a sit-alone harness fell on more difficult routes ($p = 0.004$) and sustained fewer severe injuries ($p = 0.039$). Falls on more difficult routes were associated with less severe injuries ($p < 0.001$) [82].

Indoor Climbing
For indoor climbing, Limb [26] found no correlation between injury rate and the provision of safety mats, but the mats had some influence on injury pattern.

Ice Climbing
In one study, overuse syndromes correlated positively with training hours ($p < 0.01$) [27].

Mountaineering
On 8,000 m peaks, overall death rates and death rates during descent from the summit increased with summit height [75, 80]. More people on Everest die on the descent (56%) than on ascent (10%) [75]. The faster the ascent to an altitude above 2,500 m, the higher is the prevalence of acute mountain sickness, which varies from region to region between 8 and 84%, while it is 5–15% for HAPE [83, 84].

### What Are the Inciting Events?

To trigger new safety developments the inciting events of injuries are important data. The most frequent inciting factor for injury in all disciplines (rock, ice and mountain climbing) is a fall [5, 27, 64]. Falls on more difficult routes were associated with less severe injuries [82]. Performing a strenuous move is the most frequent underlying factor in overuse injuries. In alpine mountaineering, fatigue is discussed as a very important factor which causes stumbling and falls [43]. This may explain the peak of accidents in the early afternoon and should remind the climbers to be especially careful at this time of their tour.

### Injury Prevention

Until now, little research has been performed to test the effectiveness of preventive measures.

*Traditional and Sport Climbing*

Josephsen et al. [14] found that few of the injury prevention strategies employed by boulderers were associated with reductions in the number of injuries. The incidence of these injuries was unrelated to the use of a spotter, number of spotters, use of pads and number of pads. Of the preventive measures employed, only two provided a protective effect: taping of the wrist and weight training. In contrast, finger taping, which is frequently performed to prevent pulley injuries, was ineffective in preventing injury in several other studies [14, 85–87].

Even if scientific data are sparse, general safety strategies do apply and are recommended. Based on the current state of knowledge, the following preventive measures seem reasonable: (a) spotters and crash pads in bouldering, (b) closed intersections of mats in indoor climbing, (c) dynamic belay technique, (d) proper training on belay techniques, (e) double check – partner check of knot, harness and belay device, (f) use of a helmet in alpine (traditional) climbing, (g) general recommendations of route setting in first ascents (positioning of bolts, belay chains at sport climbs, stainless steel bolts, etc.), (h) use of equipment with the UIAA safety label, (i) warm up and cool down, and (j) neglect of campus board use in young climbers before closure of growth plates.

## Further Research

Objective reporting of the injury site and its severity varied in most of these papers according to the injury definition and methodology used. This creates differences in the injury and fatality results and conclusions, which in turn makes inter-study comparisons difficult or impossible. In the absence of a common injury incidence and injury severity scoring system, some authors used the NACA score, while others used the AIS or ISS score [5, 27]. Nevertheless, all these scores demonstrated weaknesses in the evaluation of mountaineering and climbing injuries [5, 27]. Therefore a simple and common protocol was developed through a working group of the UIAA Medical Commission to report injuries in mountaineering and climbing studies [88]. These definitions should be used to allow inter-study comparison.

Further studies should address the following: (1) The use of a common score is essential and the UIAA MedCom score should be implemented in all studies. (2) Prospective studies are necessary to better evaluate cohort fatalities for the various climbing subdisciplines. (3) Predictors and preventive strategies for finger injuries must be prospectively tested and developed. (4) The influence of campus board training on the fingers must be further explored. (5) Further research is needed on the residual effects of injuries and osteoarthritis in later life. (6) Even if climbing is a regular part in rehabilitation training of other injuries, too little research is currently performed in this field. (7) Because most of the research to date has relied on self-report of injury, medical evaluation of injury is required. (8) Injury-preventive strategies must be further explored (e.g.

equipment, training of the antagonists, stretching, fall technique and training, etc.). (9) Analyses of age-related injuries (young, middle- and old-aged climbers) are missing. (10) Little information is present on beneficial effects of climbing, e.g. in older people, rehabilitation, social behavior strategies, etc. (11) Curricula for sport-specific first aid training should be developed and such courses should be offered to the climbers.

## References


1 Hochholzer T, Schöffl V: One Move Too Many, ed 2. Ebenhausen, Lochner Verlag, 2006.

2 Schöffl V, Einwag F, Strecker W, Schöffl I: Strength measurement after conservatively treated pulley ruptures in climbers. Med Sci Sports Exerc 2006;38:637–643.

3 Rohrbough JT, Mudge MK, Schilling RC: Overuse injuries in the elite rock climber. Med Sci Sports Exerc 2000;32:1369–1372.

4 Bowie WS, Hunt TK, Allen HA Jr: Rock-climbing injuries in Yosemite National Park. West J Med 1988;149:172–177.

5 Schöffl V, Morrison AB, Schwarz U, Schöffl I, Küpper T: Evaluation of injury and fatality risk in rock and ice climbing. Sport Med 2010;40:657–679.

6 Schöffl VR, Schöffl I: Finger pain in rock climbers: reaching the right differential diagnosis and therapy. J Sports Med Phys Fitness 2007;47:70–78.

7 Jones G, Asghar A, Llewellyn DJ: The epidemiology of rock climbing injuries. Br J Sports Med 2007;42:773–778.

8 Gerdes EM, Hafner JW, Aldag JC: Injury patterns and safety practices of rock climbers. J Trauma 2006;61:1517–1525.

9 Kubiak EN, Klugman JA, Bosco JA: Hand injuries in rock climbers. Bull NYU Hosp Jt Dis 2006;64:172–177.

10 Logan AJ, Makwana N, Mason G, Dias J: Acute hand and wrist injuries in experienced rock climbers. Br J Sports Med 2004;38:545–548.

11 Wright DM, Royle TJ, Marshall T: Indoor rock climbing: who gets injured? Br J Sports Med 2001;35:181–185.

12 Schöffl V, Küpper T: Injuries at the 2005 World Championships in Rock Climbing. Wilderness Environ Med 2006;17:187–190.

13 Schöffl V, Winkelmann HP: Accident statistics at indoor climbing walls. Unfallstatistik an Indoor-Kletteranlagen (in German). Sportverletz Sportschaden 1999;13:14–16.

14 Josephsen G, Shinneman S, Tamayo-Sarver J, Josephsen K, Boulware D, Hunt M, Pham H: Injuries in bouldering: a prospective study. Wilderness Environ Med 2007;18:271–280.

15 Addiss DG, Baker SP: Mountaineering and rock-climbing injuries in US national parks. Ann Emerg Med 1989;18:975–979.

16 American Alpine Club: Accidents in North American mountaineering. American Alpine Club 2006;9:59.

17 Canadian Alpine Club: Accidents in North American mountaineering, vol. 1. Canadian Alpine Club, 2005.

18 Hartsock LA, Feagin JA Jr, Ogilvie BC: Climbing and the older athlete. Clin Sports Med 1991;10:257–267.

19 Paige TE, Fiore DC, Houston JD: Injury in traditional and sport rock climbing. Wilderness Environ Med 1998;9:2–7.

20 Zafren K, Durrer B, Herry JP, Brugger H: Lightning injuries: prevention and on-site treatment in mountains and remote areas. Official guidelines of the International Commission for Mountain Emergency Medicine and the Medical Commission of the International Mountaineering and Climbing Federation (ICAR and UIAA MEDCOM). Resuscitation 2005;65:369–372.

21 Basnyat B, Lemaster J, Litch JA: Everest or bust: a cross-sectional, epidemiological study of acute mountain sickness at 4,243 meters in the Himalayas. Aviat Space Environ Med 1999;70:867–873.

22 Neuhof A, Hennig FF, Schöffl I, Schöffl V: Injury risk evaluation in sport climbing. Int J Sports Med 2011;32:794–800.

23 Nelson NG, McKenzie LB: Rock climbing injuries treated in emergency departments in the US, 1990–2007. Am J Prev Med 2009;37:195–200.

24 Schöffl V, Hochholzer T, Winkelmann HP, Strecker W: Pulley injuries in rock climbers. Wilderness Environ Med 2003;14:94–100.

25 Backe S, Ericson L, Janson S, Timpka T: Rock climbing injury rates and associated risk factors in a general climbing population. Scand J Med Sci Sports 2009;19:850–856.

26 Limb D: Injuries on British climbing walls. Br J Sports Med 1995;29:168–170.

27 Schöffl V, Schöffl I, Schwarz U, Hennig F, Küpper T: Injury-risk evaluation in water ice climbing. Med Sport 2009;2:32–38.

28 McIntosh SE, Leemon D, Visitacion J, Schimelpfenig T, Fosnocht D: Medical incidents and evacuations on wilderness expeditions. Wilderness Environ Med 2007;18:298–304.
29 Stephens BD, Diekema DS, Klein EJ: Recreational Injuries in Washington State National Parks. Wilderness Environ Med 2005;16:192–197.
30 Küpper T: Workload and professional requirements for alpine rescue; professoral thesis, RWTH Aachen Technical University, 2006 (English publication in preparation). Aachen, Aachen Technical University, 2006.
31 Burtscher M, Philadelphy M, Nachbauer W, Likar R: Alpine Notfallstatistik – Langzeitergebnisse und notwendige Konsequenzen, Todesfallrisiko beim Bergsport; in Jenny E, Flora G (eds): Jahrbuch 1994. Innsbruck, Österr. Ges. f. Alpin- & Höhenmedizin, 1994, pp 145–152.
32 Schussmann LC, Lutz LJ, Shaw RR, Bohn CR: The epidemiology of mountaineering and rock climbing accidents. Wilderness Environ Med 1990;1:235–248.
33 Carmeli E, Wertheim M: Hand injuries in young and old wall climbers. Handverletzungen bei jugendlichen und erwachsenen Sportkletterern (in German). Dtsch Z Sportmed 2001;52:285–288.
34 Schöffl V, Hochholzer T, Imhoff A: Radiographic changes in the hands and fingers of young, high-level climbers. Am J Sports Med 2004;32:1688–1694.
35 Schöffl V, Hochholzer T, Winkelmann HP, Strecker W: Differential diagnosis of finger pain in sport climbers. Differentialdiagnose von Fingerschmerzen bei Sportkletterern (in German). Dtsch Z Sportmed 2003;54:38–43.
36 Schöffl V, Küpper T: Rope-tangling injuries – how should a climber fall? Wilderness Environ Med 2008;19:146–149.
37 Schöffl V, Schöffl I: Finger pain in rock climbers – reaching the right differential diagnosis. J Sports Med Phys Fitness 2007;47:70–78.
38 Schöffl VR, Hochholzer T, Imhoff AB, Schöffl I: Radiographic adaptations to the stress of high-level rock climbing in junior athletes: a 5-year longitudinal study of the German junior national team and a group of recreational climbers. Am J Sports Med 2007;35:86–92.
39 Rooks MD: Rock climbing injuries. Sports Med 1997;23:261–270.
40 Rooks MD, Johnston RB 3rd, Ensor CD, McIntosh B, James S: Injury patterns in recreational rock climbers. Am J Sports Med 1995;23:683–685.
41 McLennan JG, Ungersma J: Mountaineering accidents in the Sierra Nevada. Am J Sports Med 1982;11:160–163.
42 Jakus PM, Shaw WD: An empirical analysis of rock climbers' response to hazard warnings. Risk Anal 1996;16:581–586.
43 Küpper T: Workload and Professional Requirements for Alpine Rescue. Aachen, Aachen Technical University, 2006.
44 Neuhof A, Hennig FF: Injury risk evaluation in sport climbing. Int J Sports Med 2011;32:794–800.
45 Schöffl V: Hand Injuries in Rock Climbing. Handverletzungen beim Klettern (in German). Dtsch Z Sportmed 2008;59:85–90.
46 Roloff I, Schöffl VR, Vigouroux L, Quaine F: Biomechanical model for the determination of the forces acting on the finger pulley system. J Biomech 2006;39:915–923.
47 Schöffl I, Oppelt K, Jungert J, Schweizer A, Neuhuber W, Schöffl V: The influence of the crimp and slope grip position on the finger pulley system. J Biomech 2009;42:2183–2187.
48 Schöffl I, Oppelt K, Jungert J, Schweizer A, Bayer T, Neuhuber W, Schöffl V: The influence of concentric and eccentric loading on the finger pulley system. J Biomech 2009;42:2124–2128.
49 Schweizer A: Lumbrical tears in rock climbers. J Hand Surg Br 2003;28:187–189.
50 Schöffl V, Hochholzer T, Schöffl I: Extensor hood syndrome – osteophytic irritation of digital extensor tendons in rock climbers. Wilderness Environ Med 2011;21:253–256.
51 Hochholzer T, Schöffl VR: Epiphyseal fractures of the finger middle joints in young sport climbers. Wilderness Environ Med 2005;16:139–142.
52 Schöffl I, Bayer T, Schöffl V: Flap irritation phenomenon (FLIP): etiology of chronic tenosynovitis after finger pulley rupture. J Appl Biomech 2011;27:291–296.
53 Logan AJ, Mason G, Dias J, Makwana N: Can rock climbing lead to Dupuytren's disease? Br J Sports Med 2005;39:639–644.
54 Hochholzer T, Schöffl V: Osteoarthrosis in finger joints of rock climbers. Degenerative Veränderungen der Fingergelenke bei Sportkletterern (in German). Dtsch Z Sportmed 2009;60:145–149.
55 Sylvester AD, Christensen AM, Kramer PA: Factors influencing osteological changes in the hands and fingers of rock climbers. J Anat 2006;209:597–609.
56 Förster R, Penka G, Bosl T, Schöffl VR: Climber's back – form and mobility of the thoracolumbar spine leading to postural adaptations in male high ability rock climbers. Int J Sports Med 2009;30:53–59.
57 Schöffl V, Popp D, Dickschass J, Küpper T: Superior labral anterior-posterior lesions in rock climbers – primary double tenodesis? Clin J Sport Med 2011;21:261–263.
58 Schöffl V, Schneider H, Küpper T: Coracoid impingement syndrome due to intensive rock climbing training. Wilderness Environ Med 2011;22:126–129.

59 Schöffl VR, Harrer J, Küpper T: Biceps tendon ruptures in rock climbers. Clin J Sport Med 2006; 16:426–427.
60 Climbing shoes – Is pain insane? (www.thebmc.co.uk/Feature.aspx?id=3156).
61 Van der Putten EP, Snijder CJ: Shoe design for prevention of injuries in sport climbing. Appl Ergon 2001;32:379–387.
62 Schöffl V, Winkelmann HP: Foot deformations in sport climbers. Fussdeformitäten bei Sportkletterern (in German). Dtsch Z Sportmed 1999;50:73–76.
63 Schöffl V, Morrison AB, Schwarz U, Schöffl I, Küpper T: Evaluation of injury and fatality risk in rock and ice climbing Sport Med 2010;40:657–679.
64 Mosimann U: Notfälle beim Eisklettern. Bergundsteigen 2006:70–73.
65 DAV: Bergunfallstatistik 2006–2007. DA eV, München, 2008.
66 Ferris BG: Mountain-climbing accidents in the United States. N Engl J Med 1963;268:430–431.
67 Hubicka E: Rock climbing injuries sustained at the training centre in Ceský Ráj (author's transl). Acta Chir Orthop Traumatol Czech 1977;44:77–82.
68 Canadian Alpine Club (www.alpineclub-edm.org/accidents/type.asp?type=ice+climbing).
69 DAV: Bergunfallstatistik 2004–2005. DA eV, München; 2006.
70 Monasterio ME: Accident and fatality characteristics in a population of mountain climbers in New Zealand. NZ Med J 2005;118:U1249.
71 McIntosh SE, Campbell AD, Dow J, Grissom CK: Mountaineering fatalities on Denali. High Alt Med Biol 2008;9:89–95.
72 Shlim DR, Houston R: Helicopter rescues and deaths among trekkers in Nepal. JAMA 1989;261:1017–1019.
73 Avery JG, Harper P, Ackroyd S: Do we pay too dearly for our sport and leisure activities? An investigation into fatalities as a result of sporting and leisure activities in England and Wales. Public Health 1990;104:417–423.
74 Malcom M: Mountaineering fatalities in Mount Cook National Park. NZ Med J 2001;114:78–80.
75 Firth PG, Zheng H, Windsor JS, Sutherland AI, Imray CH, Moore GW, Semple JL, Roach RC, Salisbury RA: Mortality on Mount Everest, 1921–2006: descriptive study. BMJ 2008;337:a2654.
76 Pollard A, Clarke C: Deaths during mountaineering at extreme altitude. Lancet 1988;1:1277.
77 Salisbury RA: The Himalayan Database: The Expedition Archives of Elizabeth Hawley. Golden/Colo, American Alpine Club, 2004.
78 Salisbery RA, Hawley E: The Himalaya by the numbers (www.himalayandatabase.com).
79 Windsor JS, Firth PG, Grocott MP, Rodway GW, Montgomery HE: Mountain mortality: a review of deaths that occur during recreational activities in the mountains. Postgrad Med J 2009;85:316–321.
80 Huey RB, Eguskitza X: Limits to human performance: elevated risks on high mountains. J Exp Biol 2001;204:3115–3119.
81 Llewellyn DJ, Sanchez X: Individual differences and risk taking in rock climbers. Psychol Sport Exerce 2008;9:423–426.
82 Hohlrieder M, Lutz M, Schubert H, Eschertzhuber S, Mair P: Pattern of injury after rock-climbing falls is not determined by harness type. Wilderness Environ Med 2007;18:30–35.
83 Basnyat B, Lemaster J, Litch JA: Everest or bust: a cross sectional, epidemiological study of acute mountain sickness at 4,243 meters in the Himalayas. Aviat Space Environ Med 1999;70:867–873.
84 Murdoch DR: Altitude illness among tourists flying to 3,740 m elevation in the Nepal Himalayas. J Travel Med 1995;2:255–256.
85 Schweizer A: Biomechanical effectiveness of taping the A2 pulley in rock climbers. J Hand Surg Br 2000; 25:102–107.
86 Schöffl I, Einwag F, Strecker W, Hennig F, Schöffl V: Impact of taping after finger flexor tendon pulley ruptures in rock climbers. J Appl Biomech 2007;23:52–62.
87 Rettig AC, Stube KS, Shelbourne KD: Effects of finger and wrist taping on grip strength. Am J Sports Med 1997;25:96–98.
88 Schöffl V, Morrison AB, Hefti U, Schwarz U, Küpper T: The UIAA Medical Commission Injury Classification for Mountaineering and Climbing Sports; in No. 17. 10.05.2010. Official Standards of the Union Internationale des Associations d'Alpinisme (UIAA), 2010:1–8.
89 Smith LO: Alpine climbing: injuries and illness. Phys Med Rehabil Clin N Am 2006;17:633–644.
90 Hearns ST, Fraser MH, Allan DB, McLean AN: Spinal injuries in Scottish mountaineers. Wilderness Environ Med 2006;17:191–194.



PD Dr. med. Volker Schöffl, MHBA
Kaimsgasse 30
DE–96052 Bamberg (Germany)
Tel. +49 95150312241
E-Mail volker.schoeffl@me.com

Heggie TW, Caine DJ (eds): Epidemiology of Injury in Adventure and Extreme Sports.
Med Sport Sci. Basel, Karger, 2012, vol 58, pp 44–56

# The Epidemiology of Injury in Hang-Gliding and Paragliding

Tiina Rekand

Department of Neurology, Haukeland University Hospital, Bergen, Norway

**Abstract**

Para- and hang-gliding are modern air sports that developed in the 20th century. Performers should possess technical skills and manage certified equipment for successful flight. Injuries may happen during the take-off, flight and landing. PubMed was searched using the search terms 'paragliding' and/or 'hang-gliding'. The reference lists of articles identified in the search strategy were also searched for relevant articles. The most common injuries are fractures, dislocations or sprains in the extremities, followed by spinal and head traumas. Multiple injuries after accidents are common. Collision with electrical wires may cause burn injuries. Fatal outcomes are caused by brain injuries, spinal cord injuries at the cervical level or aorta rupture. Accidents happen because of risk-taking behavior, lack of education or use of self-modified equipment. Observational studies have suggested the need for protection of the head, trunk and lower extremities. The measures proposed are often based on conclusions of observational studies and not proven through randomized studies. Better education along with focusing on possible risk factors will probably diminish the risks of hang- and paragliding. Large denominator-based case series, case-control and population-based studies are needed for assessment of the risks of hang- and paragliding.



The first attempts of gliding were performed centuries ago. However, a safe landing was a problem that remained unsolved for a long time. German engineer Otto Lilienthal (1848–1896) improved gliding equipment based on better understanding of the physics of flight process in the 1890s. He is considered to be the first successful aviator with multiple flights and founder of the science of aerodynamics [1]. He developed several types of gliders which were based on fundamental research on birds and airfoils. His aircraft were controlled by weight shift which inspired later constructors, but his solutions were not completely safe and his life ended with a crash at the age of 48.

During the first decade of the 20th century, stiffened flexible wings were further developed. In 1948, Francis and Gertrude Rogallo applied a kite patent for fully flexible

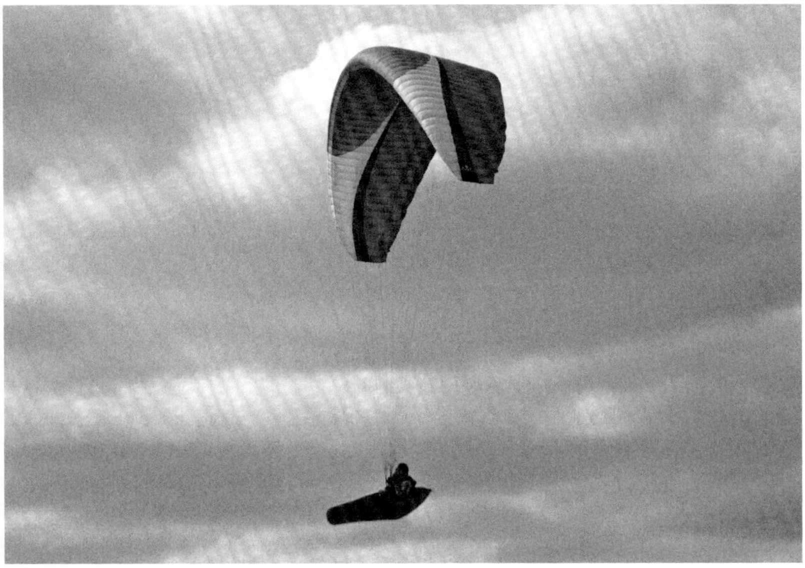

**Fig. 1.** Modern hang-glider where the pilot is fixed to a cocoon-like harness suspended from the airframe.

kited wings which became known as the Rogallo wing [2]. The modern hang-glider is a non-motorized aircraft which is made of an aluminum alloy and is controlled by shift of body weight, and the pilot is fixed to a cocoon-like harness suspended from the airframe (fig. 1). Sometimes air flight control systems are installed in the hang-glider. The hang-glider is launched from a hill slope by running against the wind to accelerate, or alternately, winches or aircraft may be used for launching.

Paragliders are developed from parachutes and are free-flying foot-launched aircraft. Parachutes with gliding abilities were developed in the 1950s. Domina Jalbert (1904–1991) invented a parafoil which had sectioned cells of aerofoil shape, an open leading edge and closed trailing edge which allowed passage through the air – the wing construction which is the basis of modern paragliders [3]. He took the patent on the equipment in 1963. The modern paraglider consists of the wing, a harness which allows sitting and instruments such as vario-altimeter, radio and sometimes GPS. Paragliders are launched by the running of pilot, but winches or motor power (powered paragliding) may be used as well. In general, paragliders are more portable and can be landed in a smaller area than hang-gliders, but the flight is more influenced by strong wind.

Although hang- and paragliding are technically different activities, both are categorized as extreme sports. The number of amateurs in the world is not known. Both hang- and paragliding are competitive sports with records in altitude, speed and length in gliding. Both sports are dependent on considerable technical skills and appropriate equipment. Both hang- and paragliding are divided into different performance levels according to pilot skills and education.

The current chapter is based on a systematic search of PubMed using the search terms 'paragliding' and 'hang-gliding'. All available studies are included. The reference lists of articles retrieved were also searched for relevant articles.

Scientific publications regarding injuries following hang- and paragliding are still limited. Therefore a systematic review of injuries has apparent limitations such as: (1) small sample sizes in many studies; (2) denominator-based data are lacking – most reports are case reports or cross-sectional studies; (3) studies are retrospective, which is not as optimal as prospective studies for assessment of epidemiological trends; (4) worldwide or national epidemiological data are missing; (5) in some studies, only one type of injury is reported which makes overview of all injuries incomplete, and (6) studies are descriptive in nature – few risk factors or preventive measures have been tested. It is important to take these limitations into consideration to interpret this overview and the findings in the studies.

## Who Is Affected by the Injury?

Epidemiological data on injuries related to hang- or paragliding have not been systematically studied in recent years. The main findings in the available studies are summarized in table 1, which reveals that hang-gliding studies consist of case series and cross-sectional surveys. Data sources include hospital records, autopsy and police reports, and reports from pilot schools. The age range, although not consistently reported, varies from 13 to 73 years. However, most participants were young adults. Injury rates, when reported, range from 0.007 to 0.08 injuries per 1,000 pilots. Table 1 reveals that studies on paragliding also consist of case series and cross-sectional studies. Data sources are primarily medical records, but also include rescue data. The age range of participants is not provided in more than half of the studies. In three studies, the age range was 15–59 years. Injury rates were not provided for paragliding.

One study from Auckland, New Zealand, studied injuries related to all parasport activities including parachuting, paragliding, parasailing and hang-gliding between 1994 and 2002 [4]. Of a total of 11,060 admissions, 38 injured persons were related to parasport activities. Paragliding was responsible for 34% of injuries. Tongue [5] studied injuries related to hang-gliding in California. He found 144 registered injuries in the period 1973–1975, 37 of them fatalities.

## Where Does Injury Occur?

### *Anatomical Location*

Knowledge of the anatomical location of injury can be vital for sports medicine staff as well as epidemiologists, helping to highlight which areas are most likely to

**Table 1.** Number and estimated injury rate after hang- and paragliding accidents

| Study | Study design | ATA source | Participants n | Age range | Injuries n | Estimated injury rate |
|---|---|---|---|---|---|---|
| *Hang-gliding* | | | | | | |
| Krissoff and Eisenman 1975 [22] | case series | MR, autopsy reports | 12 | 23–30* | 38 | not given |
| Krissoff 1976 [18] | case series | MR | 18 | 12–34* | 35 | not given |
| Tongue 1977 [5] | cross-sectional | MR, accident reports | 181 | not given | 184 | 0.08 |
| Yuill 1977 [2] | cross-sectional | BHGA | 2,461 | not given | 51 | 0.018 |
| Mang and Karpt 1977 [15] | cross-sectional | reports from the pilot schools | 3,325 | not given | 106 | 0.017 |
| Margreiter and Lugger 1978 [7] | cross-sectional | police reports, MR | 73 | 19–61 | 122 | 0.102 |
| Bell 1978 [6] | case series | MR, Q | 44 | 20–40 | 58 | not given |
| Penschuck 1980 [33] | case series | MR | 36 | not given | 60 | not given |
| Davidson 1983 [21] | cross sectional | MR | 5,000 | 13–51 | 37 | 0.007 |
| Steinke et al. 1987 [35] | case series | MR | 4 | 19–28 | 4 | not given |
| Foray et al. 1991 [34] | cross-sectional | accident reports | 200 | 13–73 | 220 | not given |
| Hasler et al. 2011 [14] | cross-sectional | MR | 181/4 | 36.3–44 | 3 | not given |
| *Paragliding* | | | | | | |
| Krüger-Franke et al. 1991 [13] | cross-sectional | Q | 218 | 15–59 | 283 | not given |
| Zeller et al. 1992 [10] | cross-sectional | Q, GBFAI | 376 | not given | 423 | not given |
| Fasching et al. 1997 [17] | cross-sectional | rescue protocols, MR, Q | 70 | not given | 79 | not given |
| Christey 2005** [4] | cross-sectional | AHTR | 38 | not given | 78 | not given |
| Gauler et al. 2006 [12] | cross sectional | MR | 41 | not given | 80 | not given |
| Rekand et al. 2009 [8] | cross-sectional/ case series | MR | 9 | 22–59 | 19 | not given |
| Hasler et al. 2011 [14] | cross-sectional | MR | 181/127 | 29–48.3 | 219 | not given |

AHTR = Auckland Hospital Trauma Registry; BHGA = British Hang Gliding Association; GBRAI = German Board of Flight Accident Investigation; MR = medical records; Q = questionnaires. * Not all reported by age. ** Includes several sports.

be injured and to assist in the direction of future preventive research. The anatomical region associated with hang- and paragliding injuries is summarized in table 2. Percent values are provided to show the relative proportion of injuries distributed by body region in each study. Because of different body positions during the flight, para- and hang-gliders are prone to injuries at different anatomical sites. Whereas upper extremity injuries appear to be more common in hang-gliders (6/12 studies), injuries involving the spine-trunk account for a larger proportion of injuries affecting paragliders (4/6 studies) (table 2). Injuries in the extremities, particularly in the lower extremity, are common in both hang- and paragliding (table 2).

Head injuries are more common among hang-gliders than among paragliders (table 2). Injuries of the spine with and without concomitant spinal cord injury have been reported as a consequence of hang- and paragliding [6–11]. Differences in location of spinal injuries may be due to different body positions during para- and hang-gliding. During paragliding the pilot sits which makes him/her prone to injuries in the thoracolumbar junction. Rekand et al. [8] surveyed spinal cord injuries following paragliding accidents in Norway and found only injuries in the thoracolumbar area of the spine. The same conclusions were made by a 10-year study from Switzerland which confirmed that fractures in the thoracolumbar area are a common consequence of paragliding [12]. Among the 37 patients with spine injuries, it was reported predominantly fractures between levels Th11-L4. Apart from thoracolumbar injuries, they reported 3 patients with spinal injury in the cervical area, 2 with mid-thoracal injury (Th5-Th6) and 2 in the sacral area in the spine. A similar pattern of spinal injuries was reported by Krüger-Franke et al. [13] in Germany and Hasler et al. [14] in Switzerland who studied 283 injuries related to paragliding between 1987 and 1989. They identified 5 injuries in the cervical area of the spine (1 of these fatal), 25 in the thoracic area (3 of these with concomitant spinal cord injuries), 61 in the lumbar area (10 of them with spinal cord injury) and 3 in the sacral area.

Christey [4] reported a predominance of lumbar injuries among all parasport injuries, among both hang- and paragliders in New Zealand. Among hang-gliders, Bell [6] reported 7 spinal injuries in the thoracolumbar junction.

Burn injuries of limbs have been described as single events, related to hang-gliding into electrical wires [6, 15, 16]. Multiple injuries are common and demonstrated in most studies (table 2).

*Environmental Location*

Environmental locations precipitating injuries are sparsely described in the literature. Both the training situation and competition may be related to injuries and are not differentiated in the literature. The optimal location and condition for hang- and paragliding are mountains with windy conditions. A change of wind direction may influence all parts of flight take-off, flight and landing [5, 6, 11, 17]. Launches from mountaintops are dangerous [18, 19]. Hang-gliders as well as paragliders are prone to

**Table 2.** Anatomical locations of injuries after hang- and paragliding

| Study | Study design | Participants n | Injuries n* | Skull/head/ brain | Spine/trunk/ spinal cord | Upper extremity | Lower extremity | Not specified |
|---|---|---|---|---|---|---|---|---|
| *Hang-gliding* | | | | | | | | |
| Krissoff and Eisenman 1975 | case series | 12 | 20 | 4 (20%) | 5 (25%) | 6 (30%) | 5 (25%) | |
| Krissoff 1976 | case series | 18 | 31 | 7 (22.6%) | 10 (32.3%) | 7 (22.6%) | 7 (22.6%) | |
| Tongue 1977 | case series | 181 | 151 | 26 (17.2%) | 24 (15.9%) | 45 (29.8%) | 33 (21.9%) | 23 (15.2%) |
| Yuill 1977 | cross-sectional | 70 | 51 | 0 | 5 (9.8%) | 15 (29.4%) | 7 (13.7%) | 24 (47.1%) |
| Mang and Karpt1977 | cross-sectional | 3,325 | 106 | 6 (5.7%) | 1 (0.9%) | | | 99 (93.4%) |
| Margreiter and Lugger 1978 | cross-sectional | 73 | 124 | 27 (21.8%) | 42 (33.9%) | 28 (22.6%) | 27 (21.8%) | |
| Bell 1978 | case series | 44 | 53 | 0 | 14 (26.4%) | 26 (49.1%) | 13 (24.5%) | |
| Davidson 1983 | cross-sectional | 5,000 | 34 | 9 (26.5%) | 3 (8.8%) | 17 (50%) | 5 (14.7%) | |
| Steinke et al. 1987 | case series | 4 | 5 | 0 | 1 (20%) | 4 (80%) | 0 | |
| Penschuck 1980 | case series | 36 | 42 | 4 (9.5%) | 7 (16.7%) | 18 (42.9%) | 13 (31%) | |
| Foray et al. 1991 | cross-sectional | 200 | 211 | 14 (6.6%) | 63 (29.9%) | 43 (20.4%) | 91 (43.1) | |
| Hasler et al. 2011** | cross-sectional | 161 | 4 | 0 | 1 | 0 | 1*** | |
| *Paragliding* | | | | | | | | |
| Krüger-Franke et al. 1991 | cross-sectional | 218 | 222 | 15 (6.8%) | 99 (44.6%) | 38 (17.1%) | 70 (31.5%) | |
| Zeller et al. 1992 | cross-sectional | 376 | 479 | 26 (5.4%) | 149 (31.1%) | 83 (17.3%) | 221 (46.1) | |
| Fasching et al.1997 | cross-sectional | 70 | 104 | 17 (16.3%) | 34 (32.7%) | 15 (14.4%) | 38 (36.5%) | |
| Christey 2005** | cross-sectional | 38 | 78 | 3 (3.8%) | 32 (41%) | 6 (7.7%) | 37 (47.4%) | |
| Gauler et al. 2006 | cross-sectional | 41 | 59 | 1 (1.7%) | 41 (69.4%) | 13 (22%) | 4 (6.8%) | |
| Rekand 2009 | case series | 9 | 15 | 2 (13.3%) | 9 (60%) | 0 | 4 (26.7%) | |
| Hasler et al. 2011** | cross-sectional | 181** | 222 | 21 (9.5%) | 129 (58.1%) | 0 | 70*** (31.5%) | 2 (0.9%) |

* Multiple injuries registered on some of participants in all studies.
** Study includes injuries after several sports.
*** Upper and lower extremity not specified.

burn injuries after crashing into electrical wires [6, 11, 15]. Collision with a tree has also been described as a cause of injury [11]. Most accidents happen after crashes in a terrain not suited for landing [4, 11, 20–22].

### When Does Injury Occur?

*Injury Onset*

Injuries caused by hang- or paragliding are always sudden-onset injuries. There are no reports of overuse injuries in these sports. However, available studies have not focused on such injuries.

*Chronometry*

The timing of injury varies by geographical location and depends on suitable weather conditions for gliding. Obviously, it is more likely that accidents will happen in warm windy weather in summer. Meteorological assessment, wind conditions in particular, is of paramount importance for a successful flight. It has been reported that most glider accidents occur between May and September during the daytime [7, 17, 20]. However, Schulze et al. [19] reported an increasing number of accidents in autumn and winter because of increased sport activity in warmer climates. For example, the most frequent accident location was California in the USA [20].

### What Is the Outcome?

*Injury Type*

Fractures in the upper and lower limbs are the most common types of injury as a consequence of para- and hang-gliding [2, 6, 7, 10]. Bell [6] reported dislocations and fractures in all parts of the upper extremities following hang-gliding accidents. Yuill [2] reported fractures of the shoulder, humerus, ulna, radius, wrist, hand in the upper extremities and in the femur, tibia, ankle and foot in the lower extremities following hang-gliding accidents in Great Britain. The studies pointed out that paragliders are at great risk for ankle injuries, obviously because of the sitting position during flights [10, 19]. Margreiter and Lugger [7] studied hang-gliding accidents in 1973–1976 in the German-speaking region of Tyrol. They identified 75 injuries, 21 of which were head traumas. Mang and Karpt [15] reported 106 hang-gliding accidents in Germany between 1974 and 1977, of which 19 resulted in severe brain injury. Bell [6] reported no head traumas in his study in the period 1974–1978 in Wales and England. He identified 2 fatal and 42 non-fatal injuries. The fatal ones suffered from retroperitoneal hematoma, rupture of the thoracic aorta and injury of the spine. Spinal cord injuries are reported after hang-gliding as well as paragliding (table 2). Because of different positioning, spinal cord injuries at the cervical level are more common among hang-gliders and the thoracolumbal level among paragliders [5, 6, 10–14]. Spinal fractures in combination with spinal cord injury are common [11, 12].

*Injury Severity*

Christey [4] reported low injury severity among parasport injuries in New Zealand. In contrast, Yuill [2] reported that 53% of hang-gliding injuries are severe such as fractures, concussions and dislocations.

Krüger-Franke et al. [13] reported that severe injuries occurred in 3% of paragliding patients and that 70% of the injured paragliders will return to paragliding. Zeller et al. [10] reported that 61% of 376 paragliding injuries required hospitalization with a mean stay of 26 days. The mean time of temporary disablement was 80 days. Only 1 injured pilot sustained a permanent neurological deficit [10]. Fasching et al. [17] analyzed 70 paragliding accidents and reported an average hospitalization of 22 days and an average working inability of 14 weeks. 34% of the injured pilots suffered from permanent nerve and joint injuries and 43% of the paragliders continue their sport despite the accident. Two pilots (11%) had another crash later. Gauler et al. [12] reported that 21 of 41 patients with spinal cord injuries related to paragliding returned to the former their workplace and place of employment. Hasler et al. [14] reported that 127 of 144 paragliders (77%) had moderate or serious injury and 18 (14%) sustained permanent neurological deficits. Among the hang-gliders, 3 of 4 were moderately or seriously injured.

*Clinical Outcome*

Hang- and paragliding are high-risk sports which may be associated with a risk of fatal outcome. Fatal accidents are caused by severe brain traumas, spinal cord injuries or aorta ruptures [2, 5, 6, 20, 22]. Studies reporting a fatal outcome after accidents are summarized in table 3, which reveals that almost all reports are of fatalities that occurred during hang-gliding. The causes and characteristics of catastrophic injuries are summarized in table 3. Among the non-fatal injuries, those of the head and spinal cord are the most serious [10]. Windsor et al. [23] studied mortality of sport activities performed in the mountains. The mortality rate related to hang-gliding was estimated to be 0.1786 per 100 participants. Unfortunately, this is the only study which reports a mortality rate.

Spinal cord injuries and head traumas are the most serious consequences of paragliding/hang-gliding accidents. Spinal cord injuries related to hang- and paragliding have been studied by Schmitt and Gerner [11]. They identified 1,016 spinal cord injuries hospitalized in Heidelberg, Germany, between 1985 and 1997. Seven cases (0.6%) were caused by hang- or paragliding. Two patients developed complete paraplegia, the others incomplete paralysis. Gauler et al. [12] showed that final outcome after spinal cord injury depends on the initial degree of bony occlusion in the spinal canal. Occlusion less than 70% indicated a favorable outcome with ambulatory function

**Table 3.** Studies reporting fatal outcome after accidents

| Study | Study design | Participants n | Deceased n | Medical causes of death |
|---|---|---|---|---|
| *Hanggliding* | | | | |
| Krissoff and Eisenman 1975 | case series | 12 | 4 | head trauma<br>aorta rupture |
| Krissoff 1975 | case series | 18 | 7 | head trauma<br>aorta rupture<br>thoracic trauma<br>cervical spinal cord injury |
| Tongue 1977 | cross-sectional | 142 | 37 | head trauma<br>aorta rupture<br>heart laceration<br>pulmonary collapse |
| Mang and Karpt 1977 | cross-sectional | 3,325 | 25 | head trauma<br>burn injury<br>multiple injuries |
| Margreiter and Lugger 1978 | cross-sectional | 73 | 7 | head trauma<br>cervical spinal cord injury |
| Bell 1978 | case series | 44 | 2 | aorta rupture<br>retroperitoneal hemorrhage<br>thoracic spinal cord injury |
| Davidson 1983 | cross-sectional | 5,000 | 1 | cervical spinal cord injury |
| Foray et al. 1991 | cross-sectional | 200 | 7 | not given |
| *Paragliding* | | | | |
| Krüger-Franke et al. 1991 | cross-sectional | 218 | 3 | head trauma<br>cervical spinal cord injury |

[12]. Katoh et al. [9] studied spinal cord injury caused by sport in Japan. A total of 528 cases were identified during 1990–1992 and 374 of these were associated with neurological deficits. Among these cases, 37 were related to sky sports and 33 sustained their injury while paragliding.

There are conflicting data about sequelae of spinal cord injuries as a result of gliding, but the sequelae depend on the anatomical level and extent of injury. Spinal cord injury at the cervical level may potentially cause permanent quadriplegia with autonomic failure of respiration, cardiac, urological and sexual function. Paragliding often causes spinal cord injury in the thoracolumbal junction [8, 12]. Paraparesis, neuropathic pain and uro-sexual disturbances may be permanent sequels of this type of injury [8, 12]. Multiple trauma may worsen the outcome after injuries [15].

*Economic Cost*
Bentley et al. [24] reviewed claim costs after injuries related to adventure tourism in New Zealand over a 12-month period. Analysis revealed that hang-gliding/paragliding/parasailing participants incurred notably greater claim costs, with 26.1% of the claims for this activity compared to just 10% of cases across all activities.

**What Are the Risk Factors?**

This review of the literature reveals few studies which have actually tested intrinsic or extrinsic risk factors. Most data are observational and conclusions are made on the basis of injury profile.

*Intrinsic Factors*
Special personality traits of hang-gliders and paragliders may precipitate accidents. The results of several studies suggest that experienced pilots tend to take greater risks such as gliding in bad weather conditions or with uncertified equipment that may cause accidents [5, 6, 10, 18]. Castanier et al. [25] studied 302 men involved in high-risk sports, among them 29 paragliders. There were no differences in personality characteristics among the studied sports (downhill skiing, mountaineering, rock climbing, paragliding and skydiving). Compared to the control persons, high-risk sport performers were more impulsive, hedonistic and insecure persons. The tests revealed negative affectivity that led them to adopt risk-taking behaviors if they use an escape self-awareness strategy [26]. The interpretation of these findings would be that bodily sensations caused by risk-taking behaviors may serve to divert the performer's attention from their ill-being and problems. Impulsive performers reported significantly more accidents [25]. Both publications point out that risk-taking behavior may be associated with socially unacceptable volitional behaviors (e.g. drug abuse, dangerous driving, etc.) as well as participating in high-risk sports [25, 27]. The study on 150 paragliders demonstrated similarities in sensation seeking between the persons with known opioid-abuse and paragliders [27].

Several studies have demonstrated that accidents occur after abuse of alcohol or drugs [5, 18, 22], while others have suggested that paragliders may have prolonged cortisol and heart rate responses compared to safe sport performers which may indicate a state of anxiety during the flight [27–29]. There are personality differences between amateurs and instructors among high-risk sport performers, including paragliders [30]. Amateurs scored significantly higher in psychoticism and self-efficacy, while instructors' scores were more like those of non-participants of high-risk sports.

*Extrinsic Factors*

The available epidemiological studies have not differentiated between participants' levels of skills; competitive or amateur participants are probably the two groups most prone to injuries [8, 10, 13, 24, 31].

There are several extrinsic factors which may relate to an increased risk of injury including experience, education, and use of protective measures and appropriate equipment. Bell [6] found that 24 of 44 injured hang-gliders were inexperienced. Zeller et al. [10] reported that the pilot's lack of experience caused accidents in 10% of cases. The importance of proper education has been pointed out in the other studies of para- and hang-gliding accidents [2, 11, 13, 15].

Several studies have pointed out that amateur-built gliders or uncertified modifications of gliders may cause accidents [5, 20, 22]. Tongue [5] found that poorly checked or experimental equipment was responsible for 9 deaths of 37 fatal accidents in California. Failure of certified equipment however is seldom the cause of accidents and was reported as the cause in 2% of all accidents by Schulze et al. [19] and 4.9% by van Doorn and Vogt [20].

## What Are the Inciting Factors?

Proper assessment of weather conditions, wind in particular, is essential to avoid accidents [2, 6, 10]. Misjudgement of wind conditions along with sudden changes of conditions may cause accidents during take-off, flight and landing phases [4, 5, 17, 20].

Several studies have pointed out that landing is the most dangerous phase of a flight [11, 13]. Landing with straight legs during paragliding is another important cause of injuries in the ankle and/or thoracolumbal conjunction of the spine [8, 10]. However, injuries are also incurred after landing on the buttocks, back or side [10, 19].

Hang-gliders are more prone to cervical and brain injuries due to their prone position during flight and landing [5]. Landing in hostile ground and uncontrolled landing after stalling are important causes of accidents [2, 4, 10].

Collision of objects in the air causes injuries during the flight, for example collision with trees as well as collisions with other gliders [11, 17]. The origin of burn injuries is often due to collision with electrical wires during the flight [2, 6, 11, 22].

## Injury Prevention

Intuitively, it seems reasonable for hang- and paraglider pilots to be required to wear safety helmets, use spine protection and wear special boots to protect ankles [4–6, 17]. However, the protective effect of such measures has not actually been tested. A randomized study design would of course be unethical. However, a case-control design may demonstrate the effectiveness of protective equipment in preventing injuries presented to the emergency department as has been demonstrated with bicycle head and facial injuries [32].

Since most accidents are caused by pilot errors, lack of training, insufficient preparation and carelessness, it follows that better education might help to reduce the risk and severity of injury in hang- and paragliding [5, 10, 19, 20, 22, 33]. Physical as well as mental fitness are important. Avoidance of alcohol and drug use before flight may prevent accidents [6]. Use of helmets, protective boots and back protection may prevent injuries [2, 6]. Proper and certified equipment is also necessary for optimal flights [4, 6, 20, 22, 33].

## Further Research

Epidemiological research on injuries sustained during para- and hang-gliding is lacking. Several areas should be covered to identify the risks of such sports activities: (1) Further epidemiological studies are needed. The risk profile for all injuries as a result of para- and hang-gliding is still unclear. (2) Most available data arise from hospital-based case series. There is a lack of comprehensive, prospective cohort studies, and studies which determine injury rates as a basis for testing risk factors. (3) There is need for more detailed research of predictors and risk factors for injuries. Both psychological and physical factors predicting injuries should be further identified. (4) Research focusing only on competition or on instructors is lacking. (5) The study of injury mechanisms should be updated. (6) Information is scarce about the effect of changes in education or introduction of new protective measures. (7) Information about the long-term outcome after injuries and factors influencing drop-out for this kind of sport is also scarce. (8) There is a need for research on the outcome after multiple injuries.

Future research will be more successful with collaboration between para- and hang-gliding organizations and with medical specialists such as neurologists, orthopedists, physiotherapists, and so forth. Common research through medical specialties and epidemiologists would reveal the incidence and distribution of injuries following hang-gliding and paragliding as well as the risk factors associated with these activities.

## References


1 Harsch V, Bardrun B, Illig P: Lilienthal's fatal glider crash in 1896: evidence regarding the cause of death. Aviat Space Environ Med 2008;79:993–994.
2 Yuill GM: Icarus's syndrome: new hazards of flight. BMJ 1977;1:823–825.
3 Kocivar B: They're not just toys anymore – kites go scientific. Popular Sci 1972;200:94, 163.
4 Christey GR: Serious parasport injuries in Auckland, New Zealand. Emerg Med Australas 2005;17:163–166.
5 Tongue JR: Hang-gliding injuries in California. J Trauma 1977;17:898–902.
6 Bell M: Hang-gliding injuries. Injury 1978;8:148–150.

7 Margreiter R, Lugger L-J: Hang-gliding accidents. BMJ 1978;1:400–402.
8 Rekand T, Schaanning EE, Varga V, Schattel U, Gronning M: Spinal cord injuries among paragliders in Norway. Spinal Cord 2008;46:412–416.
9 Katoh S, Shingu H, Ikata T, Iwatsubo E: Sports-related spinal cord injury in Japan (from the nationwide spinal cord injury registry between 1990 and 1992). Spinal Cord 1996;34:416–421.
10 Zeller T, Billing A, Lob G: Injuries in paragliding. Int Orthop 1992;16:255–259.
11 Schmitt H, Gerner HJ: Paralysis from sport and diving accidents. Clin J Sport Med 2001;11:17–22.
12 Gauler R, Moulin P, Koch H, Wick L, Sauter B, Michel D, Knecht H: Paragliding accidents with spinal cord injury: 10 years' experience at a single institution. Spine 1996;31:1125–1130.
13 Krüger-Franke M, Siebert CH, Pførringer W: Paragliding injuries. Br J Sports Med 1991;25:98–101.
14 Hasler R, Hüttner HE, Keel MJB, Durrer B, Zimmermann H, Exadaktylos AS, Benneker LM: Spinal and pelvis injuries in airborne sports: a retrospective analysis from a major Swiss Trauma Centre. Injury 2012;43:440–445.
15 Mang WR, Karpt PM: Injuries from hang-gliding (in German). Fortschr Med 1977;95:1575, 1578–1579.
16 Davidson J, Champion S, Cousins R, Jones L: Rehabilitation of a quadruple amputee subsequent to electrical burns sustained whilst hang-gliding. Disabil Rehabil 2001;23:90–95.
17 Fasching G, Schippinger G, Pretscher R: Paragliding accidents in remote areas. Wilderness Environ Med 1997;8:129–133.
18 Krissoff WB: Follow-up on hang-gliding injuries in Colorado. Am J Sports Med 1976;4:222–229.
19 Schulze W, Richter J, Schulze B, Esenwein SA, Büttner-Janz K: Injury prophylaxis in paragliding Br J Sports Med 2002;36:365–369.
20 Van Doorn RR, de Vogt AJ: Glider accidents: an analysis of 143 cases, 2001–2005. Aviat Space Environ Med 1997;78:26–28.
21 Davidson CS: Hang-gliding injuries. N C Med J 1983;44:439–440.
22 Krissoff WB, Eisenman B: Injuries associated with hang-gliding. JAMA 1975;233:158–160.
23 Windsor JS, Firth PG, Grocott MP, Rodway GW, Montgomery HE: Mountain mortality: a review of deaths that occur during recreational activities in mountains. Postgrad Med J 2009;85:316–321.
24 Bentley TA, Page SJ, Macky KA: Adventure tourism and adventure sports injury: the New Zealand experience. Appl Ergon 2007;38:791–796.
25 Castanier C, Scanff CL, Woodman T: Who takes risks in high-risk sports? A typological personality approach. Res Q Exerc Sport 2010;81:478–484.
26 Castanier C, Scanff CL, Woodman T: Beyond sensation seeking: affect regulation as a framework for predicting risk-taking behaviors in high-risk sport. J Sport Exerc Psychol 2010;32:731–738.
27 Franques P, Auriacombe M, Piquemal E, Verger M, Brisseau-Gimenez S, Grabot, Tignol J: Sensation seeking as a common factor in opioid-dependent subjects and high-risk sport practicing subjects. A cross-sectional study. Drug Alcohol Depend 2003; 69:121–126.
28 Morton DP: Heart rate responses and fluid balance of competitive cross-country hang-gliding pilots. Int J Sports Physiol Perform 2010;5:55–63.
29 Filaire E, Alix D, Rouveix M, Scanff C: Motivation, stress, anxiety, and cortisol responses in elite paragliders. Percept Mot Skills 2007;104:1271–1281.
30 Watson AE, Pulford BD: Personality differences in high-risk sports amateurs and instructors. Percept Mot Skills 2004;99:83–94.
31 Jackson AB, Dijkers M, DeVivo MJ, Pozcatek RB: A demographic profile of new traumatic spinal cord injuries: change and stability over 30 years. Arch Phys Med Rehabil 2004;85:1740–1748.
32 Thompson DC, Rivara FP, Thompson RS: Effectiveness of bicycle safety helmets in preventing head injuries. Pediatrics 2002;109:542–543.
33 Penschuck C: Causes of injury in hang-gliding (in German). Chirurg 1980;51:336–340.
34 Foray J, Abrassart S, Femmy T, Aldilli M: Hang-gliding accidents in the mountains. Report of 200 cases (in French). Chirurgie 1980;117:613–617.
35 Steinke NM, Mortensen HM, Saether J: Hang-gliding accidents in northwest Jutland (in Danish). Ugeskr Laeger 1987;149:2049–2050.



Tiina Rekand, MD, PhD
Department of Neurology
Haukeland University Hospital
Jonas Liesvei 65, NO–5021 Bergen (Norway)
Tel. +47 55975045, E-Mail trek@helse-bergen.no

Heggie TW, Caine DJ (eds): Epidemiology of Injury in Adventure and Extreme Sports.
Med Sport Sci. Basel, Karger, 2012, vol 58, pp 57–79

# The Epidemiology of Injury in Scuba Diving

Peter L. Buzzacott

School of Sports Science, Exercise and Health, University of Western Australia, Crawley, W.A., Australia

**Abstract**

The epidemiology of injury associated with recreational scuba diving is reviewed. A search of electronic databases and reference lists identified pertinent research. Barotrauma, decompression sickness and drowning-related injuries were the most common morbidities associated with recreational scuba diving. The prevalence of incidents ranged from 7 to 35 injuries per 10,000 divers and from 5 to 152 injuries per 100,000 dives. Recreational scuba diving fatalities account for 0.013% of all-cause mortality aged ≥15 years. Drowning was the most common cause of death. Among treated injuries, recovery was complete in the majority of cases. Dive injuries were associated with diver-specific factors such as insufficient training and preexisting medical conditions. Environmental factors included air temperature and flying after diving. Dive-specific factors included loss of buoyancy control, rapid ascent and repetitive deep diving. The most common event to precede drowning was running out of gas (compressed air). Though diving injuries are relatively rare prospective, longitudinal studies are needed to quantify the effects of known risk factors and, indeed, asymptomatic injuries (e.g. brain lesions). Dive injury health economics data also remains wanting. Meanwhile, health promotion initiatives should continue to reinforce adherence to established safe diving practices such as observing depth/time limits, safety stops and conservative ascent rates. However, there is an obvious lack of evaluated diving safety interventions.


Ambient pressure increases by one atmosphere for each additional depth of 10 m of seawater. Laborers working underwater in caissons while building the Eads and Brooklyn Bridges breathed air at a pressure equivalent to the ambient pressure of the depth of the workplace and high enough to repel the surrounding water. Upon returning to the surface some would experience pain and adopt a posture reminiscent of a fashionable pose known as the '*Grecian bend*'. This affliction became known as 'the bends' [1]. A century ago, the Royal Navy commissioned J.S. Haldane and colleagues to produce a set of tables prescribing time limits for each depth a diver might safely work at while teams of sailors manned compressed-air pumps to force fresh air down against the pressure of the water. Then, during the Second World War, Jacques Cousteau and Émile Gagnan invented a dual-hose regulator which allowed divers to carry compressed gas in cylinders and to inhale it at a pressure equivalent to that in which they were diving. The *self-contained underwater breathing apparatus* (scuba) had arrived. Since first appearing in the late 1940s as a recreational pursuit, scuba diving has grown steadily in popularity and, concurrently, so too has the incidence of diving-related injuries. This review considers the epidemiology of injury resulting from the adventure sport of recreational scuba diving, conventionally defined as no-stop diving with compressed gas in open water to depths of ≤40 m. Military, commercial, technical, rebreather, cave, occupational harvester and breath-hold diving are not considered here.

An electronic search was made of articles indexed by Allied and Complementary Medicine (AMED), Ovid Journals, CAB Abstracts, EMBASE, ERIC, Medline and PsychInfo using the search terms 'div$ and (fatal$ or scuba or risk or injur$)' and Google Scholar using the search terms '(diver OR diving) AND (fatal OR scuba OR risk OR injury)'. Publications were assessed for relevance to this review and either rejected, downloaded from electronic archives or acquired in hardcopy from libraries. Each publication's reference list was examined for additional potentially relevant publications and those identified were also similarly obtained. One limitation within the literature that soon became apparent was the lack of uniformity in reporting incidence and prevalence of diving injuries. In Leicester, for example, mortality incidence was given per 100,000 divers and yet divers may make any number of dives from 1 to 500 within a single year [2]. The Professional Association of Diving Instructors (PADI) cite a number of deaths over a 10-year period without stating how many member-years that period included [3] while other studies estimate the incident rate of decompression sickness (DCS) at either 1 case per number of dives or else by the number of cases per 100,000 dives. Rarely are incidence rates given per dives (or divers), per year.

## Who Is Affected by Injury?

Between 1995 and 2007 3,558 divers were treated for decompression illness (DCI) in Australia [4]. During the first 3 years of running dive tours to the deliberately scuttled (former HMAS) Swan shipwreck offshore from the south-west of Australia, a single dive tour operator documented 27,000 dives and 8 known cases of DCI, an incident rate of 29.6 cases per $10^5$ dives, almost three times higher than the Australia-wide estimate of 10.7 cases per $10^5$ dives [5]. One potential reason why these rates differ may be that the lower figure includes many dives made well within the prescribed time/depth limits while the higher figure may have resulted from divers maximizing their dive time on the shipwreck which, as Vann et al. [6] suggest in a recent review of DCS, would closer approximate the 'true' prevalence among dives made to the maximum limits. Diving morbidity studies identified during the literature search are summarized in table 1.

**Table 1.** Recreational diving morbidity studies

| Diving morbidity | Study design | Method | Period | Sample size | Number of injured | Number of injuries per 10,000 divers per year | Number of injuries per 100,000 dives |
|---|---|---|---|---|---|---|---|
| Switzerland [7] | R | Q | – | 230 | 28 | – | 25[a] |
| Australia [5] | R | RR | 2002–2006 | 1,750,000[b] | 188 | 6.7[c] | 10.7 |
| Canada [8] | P | RR, A | 1999–2000 | 146,291[b] | 14 | – | 9.6 |
| UK [9] | R | RR | 1986<br>1990 | 34,210<br>36,434 | 52<br>80 | 15.2<br>22.0 | 7.0<br>6.7 |
| UK [10] | R | Q | 1990–1994 | 2,250 | 87 | – | 19 |
| USA [11] | R | Q | – | 1,628 | 57 | – | 34 |
| Sweden [12] | R | Q | 1999 | 1,742 | 190 | – | 152 (males)<br>127 (females) |
| Okinawa [13] | R | RR, A | 1989–1995 | – | 94 | – | 13.4 |
| Saba [14] | P | RR, Q | 1999–2000 | 47,307 | 122 | 15.5 | 64.7 |
| Japan [15] | R | Q | 1996–2001 | 2,975 | 52 | 35.0[c] | 5.2 |
| Orkneys [16] | P | RR, RD, Q | 1999<br>2000 | 32,128[b]<br>36,700[b] | 8<br>18 | –<br>– | 24.9<br>49.0 |
| Caribbean [17] | R | RR | 1989–1990 | 77,680[b] | 7 | – | 9.0 |
| Western Australia [5] | R | RD | – | 27,000[b] | 8 | – | 29.6 |

R = Retrospective, P = prospective; RR = records review, RD = recorded dives; A = air fills, Q = questionnaire.
[a] Injured included recreational, military and commercial divers and 63% had a patent foramen ovale.
[b] Dives, not divers.
[c] Per 10,000 divers. It is not known how many diver-years were included.

### Where Does Injury Occur?

The protean nature of diving injuries means there is barely a location on or within the human body that is not susceptible to insult. The most common injury involves trauma to the ears and/or sinuses [18], which may not require treatment and often go unreported [19]. Of 49 confirmed cases of DCS reported to the Diver's Alert Network (DAN) in 2007, 6 (12%) included loss of bladder control and 23 (46%) included skin manifestations [19]. Of 347 medical inquiries to DAN concerning barotrauma, 212 (62%) affected the ear, 57 (16%) were related to the sinuses, 51 (15%) to the lungs, 21 (6%) to the face, 3 (1%) to the stomach, and 3 (1%) were related to the teeth [19].

**Table 2.** DCS and CAGE symptom onset time following surfacing [26]

| Time till onset | DCS (n = 70) | CAGE (n = 39) |
|---|---|---|
| On surfacing from dive | 0 (0%) | 27 (69%) |
| Surfacing to 10 min | 12 (17%) | 5 (13%) |
| 11–30 min | 14 (20%) | 2 (5%) |
| 31–60 min | 5 (7%) | 1 (3%) |
| 61 min–6 h | 13 (19%) | 1 (3%) |
| 6–24 h | 15 (21%) | 1 (3%) |
| Over 24 h | 2 (3%) | 0 |
| Unknown or unclear | 9 (13%) | 2 |
| Total | 70 (100%) | 39 (100%) |

Pressure-related injuries usually occur during descent or ascent. The genesis of DCS occurs at depth, where tissues take on additional dissolved inert gas, though physical injuries manifest following ascent when the ambient pressure drops and relative supersaturation occurs. Though more commonly associated with diving to deeper depths, the minimum depth associated with inciting DCS is merely 6 m [20]. Pulmonary barotrauma (PBT) has no such minimum depth and has occurred in even shallow training pools [21].

### When Does Injury Occur?

*Injury Onset*

A review of the records of 63 treated air divers referred to a French hyperbaric facility found the median delay between surfacing and onset of symptoms was 5 min (range 0–600) [22]. An analysis of several thousand military dives found the onset of symptoms after surfacing occurred as follows: 42% within 1 h, 60% within 3 h, 83% within 8 h and 98% occurred within 24 h [23]. Freiberger et al. [24] identified 382/2,222 (17%) cases of DCS where the first symptoms were reported either during or immediately after flying.

*Chronometry*

Examining 50 cases of sinus barotrauma, Fagan et al. [25] found symptoms developed during or immediately after descent in 34 cases (68%) and during or immediately following ascent in 16 (32%). Comparing 70 cases of neurological DCS with 39 cases of cerebral arterial gas embolism (CAGE) reported to the DAN in 1981/82, Dick and Massey [26] classified the onset of post-dive symptoms as shown in table 2. Clearly, DCS has a more latent onset than CAGE. In short, the onset of symptoms is linked to the mechanism of injury.

#### What Is the Outcome?

*Injury type*

The most common serious injuries are drowning-related, DCS and/or pressure-related, with the latter type generally classified as barotrauma, defined as '*tissue damage caused by expansion or contraction of enclosed gas spaces, due to pressure changes*' [27, p. 73]. A survey of 709 experienced recreational divers (with mean experience of 262 dives), found mild barotrauma to be the most common injury, with 369 (52%) suffering ear barotrauma, 245 (35%) sinus barotrauma, and 66 (9%) tooth squeeze [28]. 38 divers (5%) had suffered a ruptured tympanic membrane (burst eardrum), 8 (1%) a round window rupture, and 5 (1%) subcutaneous emphysema. DCS was reported by 31 divers (4.4%). DCI is used to more broadly include cases of both DCS and arterial gas embolism (AGE), between which a differential diagnosis may be difficult at presentation and irrelevant to the treatment regime of hyperbaric oxygen. Other acute injuries associated with compressed-gas diving include those caused by unsustainable gas mixtures for the depth at which breathed (inert gas narcosis, hypoxia, hyperoxia, hypercapnia, high-pressure neurological syndrome and contamination poisoning) [29–39], marine bites and envenomations [40–44], hyperthermia [45], hypothermia [46–48], and blunt force trauma (from boats, falling objects, etc.) [49, 50]. A survey of 208 diving mothers, 136 of whom reported diving during one or more pregnancies, found significantly more birth defects among children born to women who had dived while pregnant ($p < 0.05$) [51].

An Australian analysis of 859 reported diving incidents found 168 (19.5%) involved an out-of-air problem, 57 of which (35%) resulted in diver harm [52]. The distribution of types of morbidity for those 57 incidents is presented in table 3. In total, DCS, CAGE and PBT formed the majority (71%) of injuries that followed running out of air.

The annual Diving Incidents Report published by the BSAC summarizes British recreational diving fatalities, diving injuries, incidents occurring during BSAC dive trips and diver training, rescues and decompression treatments [53–63]. It should be noted that each incident is recorded in only one classification although some may equally have been classified in another category. Any diver suffering DCI was classified as DCI. Perhaps because of this among United Kingdom (UK) divers between 1998 and 2008 DCI was the most commonly reported diving injury (n = 1,245). There were a lesser number of other types of injuries (n = 632) and even fewer fatalities (n = 180). This contrasts with a survey of 304 recreational divers in Western Australia in 2005 which found DCS to be less common than other minor diving injuries [18]. Reported injuries are presented in table 4. Among 3,819 divers at Osezaki, Japan, 406 (10.6%) reported ear barotrauma, 208 (5.6%) sinus barotrauma and yet only 72 (1.8%) reported having suffered DCS [Nakayama, pers. commun., 2005].

**Table 3.** Morbidity associated with 57 out-of-air situations [52]

| Morbidity | n (%) |
|---|---|
| Decompression sickness | 24 (42) |
| Cerebral gas embolism | 10 (18) |
| Pulmonary barotraumas | 6 (11) |
| Saltwater aspiration | 4 (7) |
| Near-drowning | 3 (5) |
| Hypoxia underwater[a] | 2 (4) |
| Pulmonary barotraumas/saltwater aspiration (suspected) | 1 (2) |
| Decompression sickness(suspected) | 1 (2) |
| Not stated | 6 (11) |
| Total | 57 (100) |

[a] Rescue resulted in cerebral gas embolism.

**Table 4.** Prevalence of diving morbidity in a single year among 304 Western Australian recreational divers

| Injury | n | % | Collective type | n | % |
|---|---|---|---|---|---|
| Vertigo/dizziness | 13 | 4.3 | | | |
| Hearing loss | 9 | 3.0 | | | |
| Tinnitus | 4 | 1.3 | ear injuries | 24 | 7.9 |
| Ruptured eardrums | 2 | 0.7 | | | |
| Ear/sinus surgery | 1 | 0.3 | | | |
| Physical injuries | 11 | 3.6 | | | |
| Other (free format) | 8 | 2.7 | | | |
| Blotchy/itchy skin | 5 | 1.6 | other injuries | 27 | 8.9 |
| Tooth squeeze | 4 | 1.3 | | | |
| DCS | 3 | 1.0 | | | |

*Injury Severity*

The consequences of drowning, near-drowning and/or related complications range in severity from a full and speedy recovery through catastrophic neurologic damage to death [35, 64–67]. Barotrauma may range in severity from 'mask squeeze' with facial bruising, barodontalgia or 'tooth squeeze', ear injuries from bruising through to round window rupture, gastric injuries such as esophageal rupture, and PBT including emphysemas (subcutaneous or mediastinal), pneumothorax, up to the most serious of diving injuries; AGE, particularly the cerebral form (CAGE), a leading cause of death or drowning among recreational diving fatalities [21, 25, 67–79]. DCS, now widely accepted as attributable to the liberation of gas from solution to form bubbles in the tissues, manifests in seriousness ranging from the type I symptoms of skin rash, pain only and general malaise, through to the neurological type II symptoms of motor function impairment, loss of bladder control, sensory impairment, permanent paralysis and even, ultimately, death [72, 80–84].

*Clinical Outcome*

After a median follow-up of 54 months for 20 American males diagnosed with inner ear barotrauma, 3 (15%) had normal audiograms, 8 (40%) had some improvement but not full recovery, and 9 (45%) had no improvement since diagnosis [85]. All had returned to diving against medical advice. Among 15 consecutive cases of PBT treated in Germany, 8 (53%) recovered completely, 4 (26%) substantially, 2 (13%) had moderate recovery, and 1 (7%) recovered minimally, requiring permanent nursing care [86]. Furthermore, a retrospective review of 50 Hawaiian cases of mild DCS or serious DCI found 33 (66%) recovered completely, 12 (24%) substantially, 2 (4%) moderately, and 3 (6%) minimally [87]. These findings were similar to a study of 63 French air divers treated for suspected spinal cord DCS which found that 67% (n = 42) had fully recovered after 1 month, 8% (n = 5) still had minor symptoms, 13% (n = 8) had moderate symptoms with mild impact on daily living, and 13% (n = 8) still had severe disability with substantial impact upon daily living [22]. The odds of a substantial or complete recovery appear good among divers presenting for treatment.

*Catastrophic Injury*

Australian diving fatality reviews have been published annually since 1972 [88–95]. These reports indicate that Australia averages 10.0 recreational open-circuit compressed-gas diving deaths per year. Between 1972 and 1993 the two leading causes of death amongst the 178 scuba diving fatalities included in the reports were drowning (n = 100, 56%) and CAGE (n = 28, 15.7%) [88]. Table 5 lists diving mortality studies identified during the literature search.

Recently, the Australian Sports Commission estimates of resident participation and Queensland Government visitor activity surveys were compared to the number of scuba fatalities recorded in Australia by DAN Asia-Pacific [5]. The fatality rate in Australia between 2002 and 2006 was estimated at 0.57 per $10^5$ dives (0.7 per $10^5$ for Australian residents and 0.4 per $10^5$ for overseas visitors) [97], which was lower than estimates for British Columbia in 1999–2000 ($2.05/10^5$) [98], the UK in 2006 ($0.8/10^5$) [60], and Okinawa in 1989–1995 ($1.3/10^5$) [13]. This may be due in part to differences in sampling and survey methodology. In British Columbia, Canada, the estimated number of air fills sold by dive centers formed the basis of the denominator, in the UK a retrospective survey was conducted and in Okinawa the number of air fills sold within a military community was used. At a popular former quarry in the UK there were 7 fatalities between 1992 and 1996, during which time 238,501 divers registered

**Table 5.** Recreational diving mortality studies

| Diving mortality | Study design | Method | Period | Sample size | Number of diving deaths | Number of diving deaths per 10,000 divers | Number of deaths per 100,000 dives |
|---|---|---|---|---|---|---|---|
| Canada [8] | P | RR, A | 1999–2000 | 146,291[a] | 3 | – | 2.05 |
| Western Australia [96] | R | RR | 1992–2005 | 76,108 | 10 | 1.3[b] | – |
| Okinawa [13] | R | RR, A | 1989–1995 | | 9[c] | – | 1.3 |
| Australia[5] | R | RR | 2002–2006 | 1,750,000[b] | 50 | 0.4 | 0.57 |
| UK [5, 60] | R | RR | 2006 | 2,000,000[b] | 16 | – | 0.8 |
| UK [2] | R | RR, RD | 1992–1996 | 238,501 | 7 | 0.3 | – |

R = Retrospective; P = prospective; RR = records review; RD = recorded dives; A = air fills.
[a] Dives, not divers.
[b] Diving deaths per 10,000 all-cause mortality aged ≥15 years.
[c] Not all divers were recreational.

to dive, generating a 5-year mortality rate of 2.9 deaths per 100,000 divers [2]. Figure 1 shows the declining deaths per 10,000 memberships among British Sub-Aqua Club (BSAC) members between 1965 and 2008 [63].

The mean number of diving deaths per year among BSAC members during the last 10 years has been 1.5 deaths per 10,000 members per year, though it is unknown how many members were engaged in non-recreational (e.g. decompression) diving during this period or how many dives each member made on average. McAniff [99] published estimates per 100,000 divers per year for the USA as shown in figure 2, based upon diver population estimates derived by training agency certifications minus estimated annual drop-out from diving. These estimates were then compared with estimates by other large-scale surveys including those conducted by Diagnostic Research Incorporated (1988) and the National Sporting Goods Association (1994). McAniff's estimates were challenged by Monaghan [100] to be inflated by an overly conservative drop-out rate and he estimated the real rate to be closer to 16.7 deaths per 100,000 diver-years. Regardless, Al Hornsby [101, p. 80] at PADI recently wrote '*. . . it appears that McAniff's estimate is currently the most suitable figure for use in scientific and medical analyses that require a diver population estimate*'.

An analysis of incident reports involving diving fatalities and membership figures for PADI generated estimates during a 10-year period of 1.66 fatalities per 100,000 divers, and 0.47 per 100,000 dives under supervision of a PADI member [3]. The fatality rate among PADI dive professionals over the same 10-year period was 1.1 per 100,000 members [3]. These rates of 1.1 and 1.66 per 100,000 divers/members over

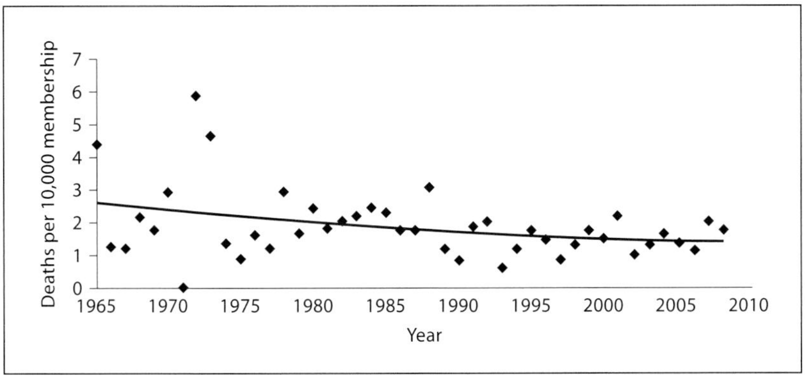


**Fig. 1.** Mortality rate among BSAC members, 1965–2008 [63].

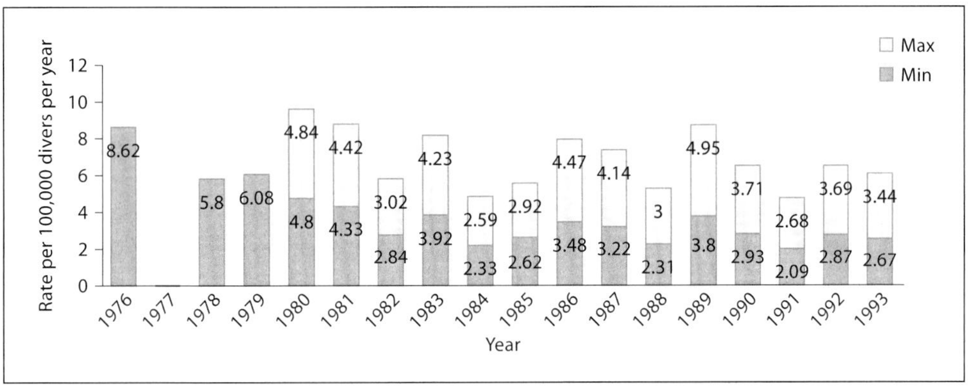


**Fig. 2.** Fatality rate per 100,000 divers per year in the USA, by year [99].

10 years could be a hundredth of that found by the BSAC if all of the divers and members were eligible for inclusion for the full 10 years (i.e. per 1,000,000 diver-years). These extremely low rates possibly reflect the increased safety associated with diving with appropriate equipment in a controlled training environment (in contrast with recreational dives made unsupervised in the open ocean).

In the United States, DAN recently compared their number of insured members against the number of dive-related deaths and, similar to BSAC, found a rate of 16.4 deaths per 100,000 member-years [102]. It should be remembered that these rates concern only fatalities that occurred during the performance of scuba diving. How the all-cause mortality rate among people who scuba dive compares with non-divers is yet to be assessed, therefore it remains unknown at this time how significantly (if at all), recreational scuba diving adds to the mortality rate of the cohort from which divers are drawn. What is apparent, however, is that fatalities involving recreational diving are extremely rare. In Western Australia there were 10 recreational diving fatalities recorded between 1999 and 2005, out of 76,108 deaths at age ≥15 years

**Table 6.** Causes of death among three recreational diving populations [106]

| Cause of death | ANZ %[a] | NUADC %[a] | DAN % |
|---|---|---|---|
| Drowning | 86 | 74 | 52 |
| Pulmonary barotrauma | 13 | 24 | 19 |
| Cardiac | 12 | 9 | 27 |
| Aspiration of vomitus | 6 | 1 | 1 |
| Trauma | 3 | 1 | 1 |
| Asthma | 2 | – | – |
| Marine animal injury | 1 | – | – |
| Coincidental | 1 | – | – |
| DCS | – | – | 1 |

[a] More than one cause of death could be nominated.

recorded in Western Australia during the same period, suggesting a rate of 13.1 recreational diving fatalities per 100,000 deaths [103]. A review of 100 consecutive Australian and New Zealand (ANZ) diving fatalities [104], 2,853 American diving fatalities reported to the National Underwater Accident Data Centre (NUADC) 1970–1997 and 83 reported in 1998 to DAN [105] found the most common cause of death was drowning (table 6).

In both the ANZ and NUADC studies, more than one cause was sometimes attributed to a single death, for example suffering PBT and drowning. Regardless, drowning is clearly the most common cause of death in all three samples. Similarly, a review of the Western Australia Coroner's Court records from 1992 to 2005 identified 24 recreational compressed-gas diving deaths, 14 of which (58%) were classed as drownings [96].

*Economic Cost*

It is not known what the average cost of such injuries is. A report into the costs of accidental near-drowning in Western Australia [107] put the average costs of a near-drowning according to the severity of the outcome, as follows: (i) moderate/severe at AUD 984,700; (ii) fully recovered (hospital admission) at AUD 6,700, and (iii) fully recovered (emergency ward only) at AUD 850.

Recent figures supplied by DAN Asia-Pacific indicate around 130 divers are recompressed for DCI each year in Australia, with an average of two treatments per diver, at AUD 900 per standard hyperbaric treatment, totaling AUD 234,000 per annum in base costs [J. Lippmann, pers. commun., December 2011]. This figure does not include afterhours call-out charges which can triple the cost of treatment because of staff call-back pay rates, nor costs associated with ambulance use or Royal Flying Doctor flights, nor extended recoveries in hospital. In rare cases, divers may even require months of physiotherapy and rehabilitation. From the above it should be clear

**Table 7.** Risk factors for running low on gas among 693 recreational dives

| Risk factor | Adjusted OR | 95% CI | p value |
|---|---|---|---|
| Surprised by low remaining gas | 21.74 | 5.00, 90.91 | <0.01 |
| Male vs. female | 13.51 | 6.41, 28.57 | <0.01 |
| Deeper average depth (per 5 m saltwater) | 3.46 | 1.85, 6.48 | <0.01 |
| Younger age (per 10 years) | 2.02 | 1.47, 2.77 | <0.01 |
| Time since last dive (per year) | 1.51 | 1.11, 2.06 | <0.01 |
| Fewer dives in last 5 years (per 100 dives) | 1.22 | 1.00, 1.49 | <0.01 |
| Higher SAC[a] (per $l \cdot min^{-1} \cdot kg^{-1}$) | 1.14 | 1.09, 1.19 | <0.01 |
| Warmth (warm vs. cold) | 4.25 | 1.28, 14.13 | 0.02 |
| Smaller cylinder volume (per l) | 1.01 | 1.03, 1.90 | 0.03 |

[a] Equivalent surface air consumption.

that diving injuries have the potential to comprise a substantial economic burden both to individuals with inadequate healthcare provisions and to health systems with finite resources.

### What Are the Risk Factors?

The influence of individual dive and diver characteristics upon the risks of running out of compressed gas were prospectively measured in Western Australia by comparing 183 dives made by divers who surfaced with <50 bar of pressure remaining with 510 control dives made at the same time and place by divers who returned with ≥50 bar remaining. The *caeteris paribus* effect of associated factors upon the likelihood of running low on gas are presented in table 7 [108].

*Intrinsic Factors*

A review of 30 Swedish scuba diving fatalities occurring between 1960 and 1976 compared the author's impressions of the predominant causes to those of other diving fatality studies of the same period [109]. Insufficient knowledge or training was the most commonly attributed risk factor (36%) [109]. When added to the proportion attributed to inadequate physical condition (12%) it appears approximately one half of the 374 fatalities (48%) were thought caused by diver-related factors rather than dive equipment or the dive environment [109]. The comparison table is reproduced here as table 8.

Comparing 101 prospective cases of DCI referred for hyperbaric treatment with 101 healthy controls, Cantais et al. [110] detected a right-to-left shunt (RLS) in 59 (58%) of

**Table 8.** Perceived causes of 374 diving fatalities in the 1960s and 1970s [109]

| | Miles (1964) UK n (%) | Webster (1966) USA n (%) | Bayliss[a] (1969) Australia n (%) | Lausche (1970) California n (%) | Unterdorfer (1974) Austria n (%) | Carlsson (1976) Sweden n (%) | Total n (%) |
|---|---|---|---|---|---|---|---|
| Insufficient knowledge or training | 83 (50) | 16 (19) | 12 (17) | 13 (43) | 2 (40) | 7 (41) | 133 (36) |
| Equipment failure | 30 (18) | 23 (27) | 12 (17) | 2 (7) | – | 5 (29) | 72 (19) |
| Inadequate physical condition | 33 (20) | 2 (2) | 6 (8) | 0 (0) | 2 (40) | 3 (18) | 46 (12) |
| Other factors | 19 (12) | 45 (52) | 41 (58) | 15 (50) | 1 (20) | 2 (12) | 123 (33) |
| Total (100%) | 165 | 86 | 71 | 30 | 5 | 17 | 374 |

[a] Bayliss did not classify the accident causes in the same way; the figures given here are only approximate.

cases and 25 (25%) of controls (OR 4.3, 95% CI 2.3–7.8; $p = 0.09$). RLS was especially associated with cochleovestibular DCI (OR 14.2, 95% CI 5.3–38; $p < 0.01$) and cerebral DCI (OR 12.9, 95% CI 4.0–42.0; $p < 0.01$). Similar prevalence of patent foramen ovale (PFO) was found by Germonpré et al. [111] when comparing 37 Belgian cases of neurological DCS with carefully matched control divers. Among the DCS divers a PFO was detected in 22/37 (59%) and in 13/36 (36%) among the controls. A meta-analysis of three combined datasets allowed Bove [112] to determine the risk of type II DCS increased 2.5 times in divers with a PFO, though the absolute risk remained relatively small (from 2.3 to 5.7 cases per 10,000 dives). A more recent meta-analysis of case-control studies found the combined odds ratio of neurological DCS in divers due to RLS was 4.23 (95% CI 3.05–5.87), which increased to 6.49 (95% CI 4.34–9.71) for divers with large RLS [113].

*Extrinsic Factors*

Whilst the association between PFO and DCS is now well established, one of the pioneering case-control studies, comparing divers with DCS ($n = 85$) to their uninjured dive buddies and other asymptomatic divers with >100 uneventful dives ($n = 91$), made a remarkable finding [114]. Wilmshurst [114, p. 35] wrote: '*Dive-related risk factors for decompression sickness (missed decompression stops, rapid ascents, post-dive ascent to altitude, dives deeper than 50 m, repetitive deep dives >40 m and frequent dives >3/day) were implicated in the majority of late neurological bends (78%) and limb bends (86%). When early neurological bends occurred, there were usually dive-related risk factors if the diver had neither shunt nor lung disease (67%) but rarely were there risk factors if a shunt was present (27%). No risk factors were present in those divers with early neurological symptoms and lung disease.*'

**Table 9.** Odds ratio for DCS by maximum depth on the last day of diving before flying [24]

| Maximum depth last day of diving | Odds ratio (n) | 95% CI |
|---|---|---|
| Depth <14.7 m saltwater | 1.00 (125) | – |
| 14.7 m ≤ depth ≤18.5 m | 1.20 (128) | 0.68, 2.10 |
| 18.5 m ≤ depth <26 m | 2.97 (142) | 1.65, 5.35 |
| Depth ≤26 m | 5.46 (140) | 2.96, 10.01 |

This suggests divers with either a shunt or lung disease are at risk of early-onset DCS even when diving conservatively but also, importantly, that dive-related risk factors for late-onset DCS are a concern for otherwise healthy divers. In a later study, Wilmshurst and Bryson [115] observed that 52% (n = 52) of divers presenting with neurological symptoms had a large or medium RLS. These findings suggest that roughly one half of all cases of neurological DCS involve dive-related risk factors. An analysis of 114 cases of DCS treated at the Fremantle Hospital Hyperbaric Chamber concluded that multi-day repetitive diving, rapid ascents, multiple ascents and flying after diving were commonly associated risk factors for DCS in Western Australia [116]. Flying after diving is known to increase the risk of DCS due to the reduction in ambient pressure. Comparing 382 cases of DCS with 245 control divers, all with known dive profiles and flight information, Freiberger et al. [24] estimated the risk of suffering DCS to increase with maximum depth reached on the last day before flying as shown in table 9.

Comparing 177 British cases of DCS with recorded meteorological changes in barometric pressure, water, air and wind-chill temperatures, wind speeds and tidal phases, Broome [117] determined that post-dive, and to a lesser degree pre-dive, air temperature was associated with increased risk of DCS.

### What Are the Inciting Events?

The most common forms of diving injuries follow running out of gas and/or ascending rapidly. Drowning was the most common cause of death among 2,404 American recreational diving fatalities between 1970 and 1992 [118]. The most common contributing factor among fatalities by the end of that review period, 1991–1992, was insufficient air (30%) [118]. This finding was reinforced by the analysis of 974 recreational open-circuit diving deaths from 1992 to 2003 which found the most common trigger commencing the series of events leading to death (41% of 346 deaths) was insufficient gas [119]. Emergency ascent then followed as the most common disabling agent, in 55% of 332 deaths where the disabling agent could be identified [119]. Factors involved in

**Table 10.** Distribution of primary contributory factors for DCI in the UK[a], 1998–2008 [53–63]

| Factor | Average number per year 1998–2008 | Total[b] n (%) |
|---|---|---|
| Depth >30 m | 36 | 394 (29) |
| Rapid ascent | 33 | 364 (27) |
| Repeat dives | 25 | 270 (20) |
| Within limits | 24 | 269 (20) |
| Missed stops | 19 | 209 (16) |
| Total[c] | – | 1,506 (100) |

[a] Approximate figures, estimated from annual summary graphs.
[b] More than one factor was credited to some fatalities in 1998, 2000 and 2001.
[c] Total without duplicate listings was 1,347 factors.

cases of DCI reported to BSAC between 1998 and 2008 are listed in table 10 (note, more than one factor may have been attributed to each case) [120]. Although diving to >30 m appeared over the period to be decreasing in prevalence as a risk factor, 27% of cases of DCI in the UK primarily involved rapid ascents, only a fifth (20%) involved dives within the accepted recreational time-depth limits and a sixth (16%) involved exceeding those limits and missing the required decompression stops.

Running out of gas is, unsurprisingly, often followed by a rapid ascent to the surface. The distribution of morbidity among an Australian sample of recreational divers between air status and type of ascent is presented in table 11. As shown, even among divers who ran out of air (n = 168), approximately equally divided between rapid ascent (n = 89) and non-rapid ascent (n = 79), a combination of running out of air and ascending rapidly had a much higher prevalence of a resultant morbidity (91%) than merely running out of air alone (9%) [52].

A probabilistic risk assessment prepared for the British Health and Safety Executive (HSE) used the prevalence of contributory factors among 849 reported BSAC diving incidents, 57 of which (6.7%) were fatal, and 277 DAN reported fatalities as a proxy for the probability of occurrence [121]. For an estimate of the likely hazard of each factor, the study used inclusion in either the BSAC incidents or the DAN fatality subsets to indicate a factor contributed to the incident or fatality. In this way each potential contributory factor was given a likelihood of being reported and a likelihood of contributing to a fatality. The top ten contributory factors associated with diving fatalities and the corresponding estimates of prevalence in the BSAC subset are provided in table 12.

The two most influential diving-technique risk factors identified in the Edmonds and Walker ANZ study (table 6) were inadequate air supply in 56% of fatalities and

**Table 11.** Type of ascent and associated morbidity for 168 out-of-air incidents [52]

| | Out-of-air type | Out of air n (%) | Morbidity n (%) |
|---|---|---|---|
| Rapid ascent (n = 89) | Octopus use[a] | 21 (12.5) | 9 (15.8)) |
| | Buddy | 14 (8.3) | 7 (12.3) |
| | Other | 54 (32.1) | 36 (63.2) |
| | Subtotal 1 | 89 (53.0) | 52 (91.2) |
| Non-rapid ascent (n = 79) | Octopus use[a] | 39 (23.2) | 1 (1.8) |
| | Buddy | 10 (6.0) | 3 (5.3) |
| | Other | 30 (18.0) | 1 (1.8) |
| | Subtotal 2 | 79 (47.0) | 5 (8.8) |
| Total | | 168 (100) | 57 (100) |

[a] Octopus use refers to using the buddy's alternate air source.

**Table 12.** Ten highest ranked potential contributory factors in 286 diving fatalities [121]

| Factor | Fatalities (n = 286)[1] | | BSAC incidents (n = 849) | |
|---|---|---|---|---|
| | n | 1 in diver-years[2] | n | 1 event in dives[3] |
| Diver separation | 126 | 11,349 | 53 | 165,094 |
| Monitor buddy | 99 | 14,444 | 25 | 350,000 |
| Brief inadequate | 83 | 17,229 | 43 | 203,488 |
| Out of air | 71 | 20,141 | 8 | 1,093,750 |
| Fail surface on separation | 65 | 22,000 | 26 | 336,538 |
| Consider consequences | 50 | 28,600 | 11 | 795,455 |
| Buddy check | 47 | 30,426 | 14 | 625,000 |
| Solo dive | 35 | 40,857 | 14 | 625,000 |
| Fail to monitor air | 32 | 44,688 | 49 | 178,571 |
| Rapid ascent | 30 | 47,667 | 101 | 86,634 |

[1] Cardiac deaths excluded.
[2] Based on an estimated annual fatality rate of 19.6 deaths per 100,000 divers and an annual average of 24 dives per diver, both of which appear higher than found elsewhere.
[3] Based on a mean 20 dives per diver per year.

buoyancy problems in 52% [104, 106]. The findings are similar to those of earlier study of 21 scuba deaths in New Zealand [122]. Differing inclusion criteria may account for the lower ranking of these factors in the HSE study (table 12), as mere inclusion within a fatality summary was assumed to imply that a factor contributed to the fatality. In the ANZ and New Zealand studies, diving medical examiners considered the

**Table 13.** Factors associated with 180 compressed-gas diving fatalities in the UK, 1998–2008 [53–63]

| Factor | Total (n = 180) $n_t$ (%)[a] |
|---|---|
| Separation | 54 (30) |
| Buoyancy loss | 50 (28) |
| Organized dive[b] | 45 (25) |
| Rapid ascent[b] | 31 (17) |
| Rebreathers | 30 (17) |
| Medical | 25 (14) |
| Out of gas | 24 (13) |
| Panic[b] | 24 (13) |
| Solo | 21 (12) |
| Equipment fail | 21 (12) |
| Seas/currents | 18 (10) |
| DCI | 11 (6) |

[a] Note: More than one factor may relate to any single fatality.
[b] Factor not classed as causal in the summary statistics but identified in the vignette.

circumstances surrounding each fatality and counted only factors deemed to have played a role in the circumstances leading up to and including the fatality. Factors associated with 180 British recreational diving fatalities that were described as *'causal'* [53–63] are summarized in table 13. There may have been other underlying triggers that led to each death and causality in an epidemiological context remains unproven. Environmental factors 'rough seas and/or strong currents' were considered relevant in just 10% of cases and diver-specific factors were limited to medical conditions and were implicated in just 25 fatalities (14%). The majority of factors associated with these 180 diving fatalities were specific to the fatal dive (e.g. separation, buoyancy loss, panic).

Supporting this view, an examination of 29 Canadian diving fatalities compared the circumstances surrounding each fatality to the Safe Diving Practices Statement of Understanding, a set of 38 safe practices prescribed by PADI [123]. In the majority of cases (86%) at least one breach of safe practices was evident and, of those, 87% of the *rule violations* were thought to have contributed to the fatality. The same method was applied to a sample of 24 Western Australian diving fatalities and certified divers were found to have broken fewer safety rules than uncertified divers (4.8 vs. 8.5, $p < 0.01$) [96]. Of the 20 divers using scuba equipment, 4 (20%) ran out of air and 2 (10%) ran low on air. There can be little doubt this was relevant to the outcome.

Annual analyses of recreational diving fatalities conducted by DAN found the three most common problems experienced by certified divers during their final dive were running out of air, buoyancy problems and/or making rapid ascents [105, 119,

124–128]. In the previous HSE study of contributing factors (table 6.11), among both fatalities and reported incidents the most frequently reported incident (n = 101/849) was a rapid ascent, though no measured rate of ascent was specified [121]. Of the 34 fatal breath-hold embolisms examined in that study, 13 (38%) involved rapid ascents and 10 of those 13 (77%) were deemed due to running out of air. The report concluded [121, p. 26]: '*The statistics show that: (i) rapid ascent is the most frequently reported contributory cause of incident, and (ii) air embolism is the second most frequent principal cause of fatality.*'

The most frequent principal cause of fatality, however, was entrapment/entanglement, for example underneath ice or inside shipwrecks. Following on from this report, Cranfield University was commissioned by HSE to conduct a research report entitled Formal Risk Identification in Professional SCUBA (FRIPS) [129]. The authors used both Fault Tree Analysis (FTA), '*. . .to show the importance of human factors to the ultimate safety of divers*' [129, p. 2] and the predictive model, Failure Mode and Effects Criticality Analysis '*. . .to demonstrate how a formal risk assessment can be carried out on SCUBA hardware*' [129, p. 2]. Using Boolean OR and AND options, FTA is most useful when aiming to identify proximate causes [130]. Similar methods have been employed by DAN in the USA [119, 131] and in Australia [95]. As with the earlier HSE report, in the FRIPS analysis scuba deaths were deemed most often attributable to drowning due to running out of air or embolism after either a loss of buoyancy control or rapid ascent. Among living, adult recreational divers these three factors have been investigated using a case-control study design both retrospectively [132] and prospectively [108].

### Injury Prevention

Though DCS, drowning and near-drowning appear to be relatively rare events, public health injury prevention initiatives have potential to reduce the economic burden to healthcare providers, potential that remains largely untapped. A study by DAN examined the probability of DCS among the recorded dive profiles of 100 cases of DCS and found that, in most cases, the dive profiles were within recommended limits [133]. These cases were then compared with 50 cases of experimentally induced DCS and to the profiles of 50,000 recreational dives with symptom-free outcomes. The authors concluded: '*The incidence of DCS in low-risk dives may not be possible to reduce further by controlling the depth-time exposure only*' [133, p. 187]. This suggests two avenues for improving diver safety; identifying additional risk factors associated with probability of DCS and increasing the proportion of recreational divers who are mindful of empirically established relatively-safe depth-time profile limits, including ascent rate. Among Western Australian scuba diving fatalities it was found that uncertified (or self-trained) scuba divers both breach significantly more established safe diving practices (4.8 vs. 8.5, $p < 0.01$) and account for 30% of all diving fatalities where the training status is known [96]. Uncertified divers have elsewhere been found to report significantly more diving injuries than certified divers (RR = 1.31, 95% CI 1.16–1.48; $p < 0.001$) [134] yet in many countries there is no requirement for self-trained divers, (who are more likely to suffer an injury and yet who may still expect treatment at the expense of the local healthcare system), to undertake any form of diving skills assessment. This is surely one area in which minor regulatory changes might assist the most vulnerable divers underwater, by requiring every diver to master even just basic diving skills, such as those endorsed in a memorandum of understanding by the Recreational Scuba Training Council, a global affiliation of diver training agencies. Meanwhile, governments continue to sell fishing licenses to untrained and uncertified recreational divers [96].

Despite repeated calls for regular health assessments by doctors with training in dive medicine, there is little evidence that either periodic dive medicals or the exclusive use of physicians trained in diving physiology offer any tangible risk reduction. The current international standard requires dive-course candidates to complete a self-assessment questionnaire and to undertake a dive medical if answering in the affirmative to any known medical contraindications. Routine screening for PFO is considered unwarranted for recreational diving as the absolute risk of type II DCS is small [113], even with a PFO (5.7 cases per 10,000 dives) [112]. Once certified, divers are rarely required to undertake subsequent diving fitness assessments. The medical fraternity should not be relied upon to reduce diving morbidity. Public health promotion initiatives have far greater potential effect although there is a dearth of health economics research into the burden of diving injuries and hard data remains sorely needed to justify greater investment in diving safety initiatives.

## Further Research

To date, the majority of diving injury studies are case-series designs, considered a '*primitive form of case-control study – one in which the controls are only implied*' [120, p. 54]. Notable exceptions are case-control studies investigating either environmental factors associated with DCS [117], physiological risk factors for DCS and PBT such as RLS and small airways disease [86, 113–115], and hyperbaric chamber experiments [135]. Larger, prospective cohort studies, though more expensive and time consuming, are needed to quantify the potential long-term effects of diving, both among those treated for diving injuries and the apparently asymptomatic [136]. Only then will divers have an accurate estimate of the risks they assume when returning to the underwater realm. Till these occur, we rely on physiological inferences and inconclusive, often controversial evidence, for example concerning the relative risk of PBT associated with asthma, the prevalence of brain damage in otherwise symptom-free recreational divers or the potential influence of gender on susceptibility of DCS. It is also recommended that future research uniformly report injury prevalence using the denominators 'per 10,000 divers' and/or 'per 100,000 dives', and incidence rates of 'per 10,000 divers per year' and/or 'per 100,000 dives per year'. From a population health perspective, the widest gap in our understanding of diving injuries awaits evaluated diving safety initiatives, which are sorely lacking. A wealth of knowledge concerning recreational scuba diving injuries has been compiled during the last half a century, more still has been studied and yet, to date, even more again remains to be discovered.

## References


1 Butler W: Caisson disease during the construction of the Eads and Brooklyn Bridges: a review. Undersea Hyperb Med 2004;31:445–459.

2 Hart AJ, White SA, Conboy PJ, Bodiwala G, Quinton D: Open water scuba diving accidents at Leicester: five years' experience. J Accid Emerg Med 1999; 16:198–200.

3 Kinsella J: The data tell us. Undersea J 2011;first qtr:80–81.

4 Lippmann J: Reviewing diving safety in Australia; in Sharp M, Franklin R (eds): 2008 Australian Water Safety Conference Proceedings. Australian Water Safety Council, 2008, pp 27–29.

5 Lippmann J: Review of scuba diving fatalities and decompression illness in Australia. Diving Hyperb Med 2008;38:71–78.

6 Vann R, Butler FK, Mitchell SJ, Moon RE: Decompression illness. Lancet 2011;377:153–164.

7 Torti SR, Billinge M, Schwerzmann M, Vogel R, Zbinden R, Windecker S, Seiler C: Risk of decompression illness among 230 divers in relation to the presence and size of patent foramen ovale. Eur Heart J 2004;25:1014–1020.

8 Ladd G, Stepan V, Stevens L: The Abacus Project: establishing the risk of recreational scuba death and decompression illness. South Pacific Underwater Med Soc J 2002;32:124–128.

9 Wilmshurst PT, Allen A, Parish T: Incidence of decompression illness in amateur scuba divers. Health Trends 1994;26:116–118.

10 St Leger Dowse M, Bryson P, Gunby A, Fife W: Comparative data from 2,250 male and female sports divers: diving patterns and decompression sickness. Aviat Space Environ Med 2002;73:743–749.

11 Dear G, Uguccioni D, Dovenbarger J, Thalmann ED, Cudahy E, Hanson E: Estimated DCI incidence in a select group of recreational divers. Undersea Hyperb Med 1999;26(suppl):abstr 34.

12 Hagberg M, Ornhagen H: Incidence and risk factors for symptoms of decompression sickness among male and female dive masters and instructors – a retrospective cohort study. Undersea Hyperb Med 2003;30:93–102.

13 Arness MK: Scuba decompression illness and diving fatalities in an overseas military community. Aviat Space Environ Med 1997;68:325–333.

14 LeFevre CA: Incidence and risk factors for decompression sickness on Saba, Netherlands-Antilles: a prospective study; thesis, University of Saba School of Medicine, 2003.

15 Nakayama H, Shibayama M, Yamami N, Togawa S, Takahashi M, Mano Y: Decompression sickness and recreational scuba divers. Emerg Med J 2003;20: 332–334.

16 Trevett AJ, Forbes R, Rae CK, Sheehan C, Ross J, Watt SJ, Stephenson R: Diving accidents in sports divers in Orkney waters. Scott Med J 2001;46:176–177.

17 Gilliam B: Evaluation of decompression sickness incidence in multi-day repetitive diving for 77,680 sport dives. South Pacific Underwater Med Soc J 1992;22:24–30.

18 Buzzacott P: Diving injuries amongst Western Australian scuba course graduates; thesis, School of Population Health, University of Western Australia Medicine, 2006.

19 Pollock N, Dunford R, Denoble P, Dovenbarger J, Caruso JL: Report on Decompression Illness, Diving Fatalities and Project Dive Exploration, 2008 Edition (based on 2006 data). Durham/NC, Divers Alert Network, 2001.

20 Van Liew HD, Flynn ET: Direct ascent from air and $N_2$-$O_2$ saturation dives in humans: DCS risk and evidence of a threshold. Undersea Hyperb Med 2005;32:409–419.

21 Raymond L: Pulmonary barotrauma and related events in divers. Chest 1995;107:1648–1652.

22 Gempp E, Blatteau J: Risk factors and treatment outcome in scuba divers with spinal cord decompression sickness. J Crit Care 2010;25:236–242.

23 Navy Department: US Navy Diving Manual. Revision 6. Naval Sea Systems Command. Washington, US Navy, 2008.

24 Freiberger JJ, Denoble PJ, Pieper CF, Uguccioni DM, Pollock NW, Vann RD: The relative risk of decompression sickness during and after air travel following diving. Aviat Space Environ Med 2002;73: 980–984.

25 Fagan P, McKenzie B, Edmonds C: Sinus barotrauma in divers. Ann Otol Rhinol Laryngol 1976;85:61–64.
26 Dick AP, Massey EW: Neurologic presentation of decompression sickness and air embolism in sport divers. Neurology 1985;35:667–671.
27 Edmonds C: Ear barotrauma; in Edmonds C, Lowry C, Pennefather J, Walker R (eds): Diving and Subaquatic Medicine. London, Arnold, 2002, pp 73–91.
28 Taylor DM, O'Toole, Ryan CM: Experienced scuba divers in Australia and the United States suffer considerable injury and morbidity. Wilderness Environ Med 2003;14:83–88.
29 Lowry C: Inert gas narcosis; in Edmonds C, Lowry C, Pennefather J, Walker R (eds): Diving and Subaquatic Medicine. London, Arnold, 2002, pp 183–193.
30 Lowry C: Oxygen toxicity; in Edmonds C, Lowry C, Pennefather J, Walker R (eds): Diving and Subaquatic Medicine. London, Arnold, 2002, pp 207–222.
31 Lowry C: High-pressure neurological syndrome; in Edmonds C, Lowry C, Pennefather J, Walker R (eds): Diving and Subaquatic Medicine. London, Arnold, 2002, pp 243.
32 Edmonds C: Hypoxia; in Edmonds C, Lowry C, Pennefather J, Walker R (eds): Diving and Subaquatic Medicine. London, Arnold, 2002, pp 195–206.
33 Edmonds C: Carbon dioxide toxicity; in Edmonds C, Lowry C, Pennefather J, Walker R (eds): Diving and Subaquatic Medicine. London, Arnold, 2002, pp 223–231.
34 Pennefather J: Breathing gas contamination; in Edmonds C, Lowry C, Pennefather J, Walker R (eds): Diving and Subaquatic Medicine. London, Arnold, 2002, pp 233–241.
35 Dickey LS: Diving Injuries. J Emerg Med 1984;1: 249–262.
36 Bennett P: Inert gas narcosis and high-pressure nervous syndrome; in Bove AA (ed): Bove and Davis' Diving Medicine. Philadelphia, Saunders, 2004, pp 225–239.
37 Clark JM, Thorn SR: Toxicity of oxygen, carbon dioxide, and carbon monoxide; in Bove AA (ed): Bove and Davis' Diving Medicine. Philadelphia, Saunders, 2004, pp 241–259.
38 Youngblood DG, Wolfe WG: Unearthly atmospheres: some dangerous aspects of diving gases; in Strauss RH (ed): Diving Medicine. New York, Grune & Stratton, 1976, pp 145–155.
39 Bennett P: The physiology of nitrogen narcosis and the high pressure nervous syndrome; in Strauss RH (ed): Diving Medicine. New York, Grune & Stratton, 1976, pp 157–180.
40 Edmonds C: Marine animal injuries; in Bove AA (ed): Bove and Davis' Diving Medicine. Philadelphia, Saunders, 2004, pp 287–318.
41 Edmonds C: Venomous marine animals; in Edmonds C, Lowry C, Pennefather J, Walker R (eds): Diving and Subaquatic Medicine. London, Arnold, 2002, pp 335–351.
42 Edmonds C: Dangerous Marine Creatures. Flagstaff/AZ, Best Publishing Co, 1995.
43 Auerbach PS: A Medical Guide to Hazardous Marine Life, ed 3. Flagstaff/AZ, Best Publishing Co, 1997.
44 Halstead BW: Hazardous marine life; in Strauss RH (ed): Diving Medicine. New York, Grune & Stratton, 1976, pp 227–255.
45 Pennefather J: Thermal problems and solutions; in Edmonds C, Lowry C, Pennefather J, Walker R (eds): Diving and Subaquatic Medicine. London, Arnold, 2002, pp 289–292.
46 Pennefather J: Cold and hypothermia; in Edmonds C, Lowry C, Pennefather J, Walker R (eds): Diving and Subaquatic Medicine. London, Arnold, 2002, pp 293–304.
47 Tipton MJ, Mekjavic IB, Golden FSC: Hypothermia; in Bove AA (ed): Bove and Davis' Diving Medicine. Philadelphia, Saunders, 2004, pp 261–273.
48 Cooper KE: Hypothermia; in Strauss RH (ed): Diving Medicine. New York, Grune & Stratton, 1976, pp 211–225.
49 Edmonds C: Trauma from marine creatures; in Edmonds C, Lowry C, Pennefather J, Walker R (eds): Diving and Subaquatic Medicine. London, Arnold, 2002, pp 325–334.
50 Sharpe A: Shark down under: shark attacks in Australian waters. Crows Nest/NSW, Kingsclear Books, 1993.
51 Bolton ME: Scuba diving and fetal well-being: a survey of 208 women. Undersea Biomed Res 1980;7: 183–189.
52 Acott C: Diving incidents – errors divers make; in Safe Limits: An International Dive Symposium. Cairns, Division of Workplace Health and Safety, 1994.
53 Cumming B: NDC Diving Incidents Report. South Wirral, Cheshire, British Sub-Aqua Club, 1998.
54 Cumming B: NDC Diving Incidents Report. South Wirral, Cheshire, British Sub-Aqua Club, 1999.
55 Cumming B: NDC Diving Incidents Report. South Wirral, Cheshire, British Sub-Aqua Club, 2000.
56 Cumming B: NDC Diving Incidents Report. South Wirral, Cheshire, British Sub-Aqua Club, 2001.

57 Cumming B: NDC Diving Incidents Report. South Wirral, Cheshire, British Sub-Aqua Club, 2002.
58 Cumming B: NDC Diving Incidents Report. South Wirral, Cheshire, British Sub-Aqua Club, 2003.
59 Cumming B: NDC Diving Incidents Report. South Wirral, Cheshire, British Sub-Aqua Club, 2005.
60 Cumming B: NDC Diving Incidents Report. South Wirral, Cheshire, British Sub-Aqua Club, 2006.
61 Cumming B: NDC Diving Incidents Report. South Wirral, Cheshire, British Sub-Aqua Club, 2007.
62 Cumming B: NDC Diving Incidents Report. South Wirral, Cheshire, British Sub-Aqua Club, 2004.
63 Cumming B: NDC Diving Incidents Report. South Wirral, Cheshire, British Sub-Aqua Club, 2008.
64 Edmonds C: Drowning syndromes: drowning; in Edmonds C, Lowry C, Pennefather J, Walker R (eds): Diving and Subaquatic Medicine. London, Arnold, 2002, pp 249–256.
65 Zwingelberg KM, Green JW, Powers K: Primary causes of drowning and near drowning in scuba diving. Physician Sports Med 1986;14:145–151.
66 Neuman TS: Near drowning; in Bove AA (ed): Bove and Davis' Diving Medicine. Philadelphia, Saunders, 2004, pp 275–286.
67 Miles S, Mackay DE: Underwater Medicine, ed 4. London, Adlard Coles Ltd, 1976.
68 Walker R: Pulmonary barotrauma; in Edmonds C, Lowry C, Pennefather J, Walker R (eds): Diving and Subaquatic Medicine. London, Arnold, 2002, pp 55–71.
69 Gallagher TJ: Scuba diving accidents: decompression sickness, air embolism. J Florida Med Assoc 1997;84:446–451.
70 Wilson HL: Otolaryngologic problems of skin and scuba diving. Arch Otolaryngol Head Neck Surg 1972;96:407–411.
71 Duffner GJ: Scuba diving injuries. Predisposing causes and prevention. JAMA 1961;175:375.
72 Boettger ML: Scuba diving emergencies: pulmonary overpressure accidents and decompression sickness. Ann Emerg Med 1983;12:563–567.
73 Becker GD, Parell GJ: Barotrauma of the ears and sinuses after scuba diving. Eur Arch Otorhinolaryngol 2001;258:159–163.
74 Becker GD, Parell GJ: Otolaryngologic aspects of scuba diving. Otolaryngol Head Neck Surg 1979; 87:569–572.
75 Freeman P, Tonkin J, Edmonds C. Rupture of the round window membrane in inner ear barotrauma. Arch Otolaryngol Head Neck Surg 1974;99:437–442.
76 Smith FR: Air embolism as a cause of death in scuba diving in the Pacific Northwest. Dis Chest 1967; 52:15–20.
77 Neuman TS: Pulmonary barotrauma; in Bove AA (ed): Bove and Davis' Diving Medicine. Philadelphia, Saunders, 2004, pp 185–193.
78 Hunter SE, Farmer JCJ: Ear and sinus problems in diving; in Bove AA (ed): Bove and Davis' Diving Medicine. Philadelphia, Saunders, 2004, pp 431–460.
79 Farmer JC, Thomas WG: Ear and sinus problems in diving; in Strauss RH (ed): Diving Medicine. New York, Grune & Stratton, 1976, pp 109–132.
80 Walker R: Decompression sickness: clinical; in Edmonds C, Lowry C, Pennefather J, Walker R (eds): Diving and Subaquatic Medicine. London, Arnold, 2002, pp 137–150.
81 Farmer JC, Thomas WG, Youngblood DG, Bennett PB: Inner ear decompression sickness. Laryngoscope 1976;86:1315–1327.
82 Rivera JC: Decompression sickness among divers; an analysis of 935 cases. Washington, US Navy Experimental Diving Unit, 1963.
83 Francis TJ, Mitchell SJ: Pathophysiology of decompression sickness; in Bove AA (ed): Bove and Davis' Diving Medicine. Philadelphia, Saunders, 2004, pp 165–183.
84 Strauss RH: Decompression sickness; in Strauss RH (ed): Diving Medicine. New York, Grune & Stratton, 1976, pp 63–80.
85 Parell GJ, Becker GD: Inner ear barotrauma in scuba divers: a long-term follow-up after continued diving. Arch Otolaryngol Head Neck Surg 1993; 119:455.
86 Tetzlaff K, Reuter M, Leplow B, Heller M, Bettinghausen E: Risk factors for pulmonary barotrauma in divers. Chest 1997;112:654–659.
87 Kizer K: Delayed treatment of dysbarism. JAMA 1982;247:2555–2558.
88 Walker D: Report on Australian Diving Deaths 1972–1993. Melbourne, J.L. Publications, 1998.
89 Walker D: Report on Australian Diving Deaths 1994–1998. Ashburton/Vic, Divers Alert Network (DAN) SE Asia-Pacific Ltd, 2002.
90 Walker D: Provisional report on diving-related fatalities in Australian waters 1999. South Pacific Underwater Med Soc J 2005;35:183–193.
91 Walker D: Provisional report on diving-related fatalities in Australian waters 2000. Diving Hyperb Med 2006;36:62–71.
92 Walker D: Provisional report on diving-related fatalities in Australian waters 2001. Diving Hyperb Med 2006;36:122–138.
93 Walker D: Provisional report on diving-related fatalities in Australian waters 2002. Diving Hyperb Med 2008;38:8–28.

94 Walker D, Lippmann J: Provisional report on diving-related fatalities in Australian waters 2003. Diving Hyperb Med 2009;39:4–19.
95 Walker D, Lippmann J, Lawrence C, Houston J, Fock A: Provisional report on diving-related fatalities in Australian waters 2004. Diving Hyperb Med 2009;39:138–161.
96 Buzzacott P, Rosenberg M, Pikora T: Western Australian recreational scuba diving fatalities, 1992–2005. ANZ J Public Health 2009;33:212–214.
97 Lippmann J: Scuba fatality rate in Australia, 2002–2006; in Recreational Diving Fatalities. Proc Divers Alert Network 2010, April 8–10 Workshop. Durham/NC, Divers Alert Network, 2011.
98 Ladd G, Stepan V, Stevens L: New method for counting recreational scuba dives establishes risk of death and DCI injury. Undersea Hyperb Med 2002;29:93.
99 McAniff J: An analysis of recreational, technical and occupational populations and fatality rates in the United States, 1970–1994. Santa Ana/CA, Professional Association of Diving Instructors, 1995.
100 Monaghan R: The risks of sport diving. South Pacific Underwater Med Soc J 1988;18:53–60.
101 Hornsby A: Models for estimating the diver population of the United States: AN assessment. Undersea J 2010;4th qtr:78–80.
102 Denoble P, Pollock NW, Vaithiyanathan P, Caruso JL, Dovenbarger JA, Vann RD: Scuba injury death rate among DAN members. Diving Hyperb Med 2008;38:182–188.
103 Australian Bureau of Statistics: Deaths. Canberra, Australian Bureau of Statistics, 2009.
104 Edmonds C, Walker D: Scuba diving fatalities in Australia and New Zealand: the human factor. South Pacific Underwater Med Soc J 1989;19:94–104.
105 Vann RD, Uguccioni DM: Report on Decompression Illness, Diving Fatalities and Project Dive Exploration, 2000 Edition (based on 1998 data). Durham/NC, Divers Alert Network, 2000.
106 Edmonds C: Why divers die: the facts and the figures; in Edmonds C, Lowry C, Pennefather J, Walker R (eds): Diving and Subaquatic Medicine. London, Arnold, 2002, pp 473–489.
107 Hendrie D: The costs of accidental drowning and near-drowning in Western Australia. Perth, University of Western Australia, 2004.
108 Buzzacott P, Rosenberg M, Heyworth J, Pikora T: Risk factors for running low on gas in recreational divers in Western Australia. Diving Hyperb Med 2011;41:85–89.
109 Carlsson K, Lidholm SO, Maehly AC: Scuba diving accidents in Sweden 1960–1976. Forensic Sci 1978; 11:93–108.
110 Cantais E, Louge P, Suppini A, Foster PP, Palmier B: Right-to-left shunt and risk of decompression illness with cochleovestibular and cerebral symptoms in divers: case-control study in 101 consecutive dive accidents. Crit Care Med 2003;31:84–88.
111 Germonpré P, Dendale P, Unger P, Balestra C: Patent foramen ovale and decompression sickness in sports divers. J Appl Physiol 1998;84:1622–1626.
112 Bove AA: Risk of decompression sickness with patent foramen ovale. Undersea Hyperb Med 1998; 25:175–178.
113 Lairez O, Cournot M, Minville V, Roncalli J, Austruy J, Elbaz M, Galinier M, Carrie D: Risk of neurological decompression sickness in the diver with a right-to-left shunt: literature review and meta-analysis. Clin J Sport Med 2009;19:231–235.
114 Wilmshurst PT: Analysis of decompression accidents in amateur divers. Prog Underwater Sci 1990; 15:31–37.
115 Wilmshurst P, Bryson P: Relationship between the clinical features of neurological decompression illness and its causes. Clin Sci 2000;99:65–75.
116 Oxer H: Safe limits – assessing the risks; in Safe Limits. An international Dive Symposium. Cairns, QLD Division of Workplace Health and Safety 1994, pp 86–92.
117 Broome JR: Climatic and environmental factors in the aetiology of decompression sickness in divers. J R Nav Med Serv 1993;79:68–74.
118 Richardson D: Reflections on diver fatality and safety statistics. South Pacific Underwater Med Soc J 1994;24:157–161.
119 Denoble PJ, Caruso JL, Dear GL, Pieper CF, Vann RD: Common causes of open-circuit recreational diving fatalities. Undersea Hyperb Med 2008;35: 393–406.
120 Cummings P, Weiss NS: Case series and exposure series: the role of studies without controls in providing information about the etiology of injury or disease. Inj Prev 1998;4:54–57.
121 Health and Safety Executive: Paras, Scuba Diving. A Quantitative Risk Assessment. Newport/Isle of Wight, Health and Safety Executive, 1997.
122 Lewis PRF: Skin diving fatalities in New Zealand. NZ Med J 1979;89:472–475.
123 Lagache E: Semiqualitative methods for scuba accident analysis. Berkley/CA, Recreational Scuba Diving Socio-Cultural Research Group, 1992.
124 Dovenbarger J: Report on Diving Accidents and Fatalities, 1996 Edition (based on 1994 data). Durham/NC, Divers Alert Network, 1996.
125 Vann RD, Uguccioni DM: Report on Decompression Illness, Diving Fatalities and Project Dive Exploration, 2001 Edition (based on 1999 data). Durham/NC, Divers Alert Network, 2001.

126 Vann RD, Denoble P, Uguccioni DM, Freiberger JJ, Perkins R, Reed W, Dovenbarger J, Caruso JL: Report on Decompression Illness, Diving Fatalities and Project Dive Exploration, 2002 Edition (based on 2000 data). Durham/NC, Divers Alert Network, 2002.
127 Vann RD, Denoble P, Uguccioni DM, Freiberger JJ, Reed W, Dovenbarger J, Caruso JL, Duncan R, Hyatt W: Report on Decompression Illness, Diving Fatalities and Project Dive Exploration, 2003 Edition (based on 2001 data). Durham/NC, Divers Alert Network, 2003.
128 Vann RD, Denoble PJ, Uguccioni DM, Freiberger JJ, Forbes R, Pieper CF: Incidence of decompression sickness in four recreational diving population samples. Undersea Hyperb Med 2004;31:304–305.
129 Tetlow S: Formal Risk Identification in Professional Scuba (FRIPS). Cranfield, Cranfield University, 2006.
130 McKee J (ed): Root Cause Analysis in Healthcare, ed 3. Chicago, Joint Commission Resources, 2005.
131 Buzzacott P, Zeigler E, Denoble P, Vann R: American cave diving fatalities 1969–2007. Int J Aquat Res Educ 2009;3:162–177.
132 Buzzacott P, Denoble P, Dunford R, Vann R: Dive problems and risk factors for diving morbidity. Diving Hyperb Med 2009;39:205–209.
133 Denoble P, Vann R, Dunford R: Predicted probability and severity of symptoms in 100 documented cases of decompression sickness in recreational diving; in Third Conference US-Japan Panel on Aerospace, Diving Physiology & Technology and Hyperbaric Medicine (UJNR). Durham/NC, Undersea Hyperbaric Medical Society, 2009.
134 Beckett A, Kordick MF: Risk factors for dive injury: a survey study. Res Sports Med 2007;15:201–211.
135 Buhlmann AA: Decompression after repeated dives. Undersea Biomed Res 1987;14:59–66.
136 McQueen D, Kent G, Murrison A: Self-reported long-term effects of diving and decompression illness in recreational scuba divers. Br J Sports Med 1994;28:101–104.

Peter L. Buzzacott, PhD
Research Associate, School of Sports Science, Exercise and Health
The University of Western Australia
M408, 35 Stirling Highway, Crawley, WA 6009 (Australia)
Tel. +61 8 6488 3842, E-Mail peter.buzzacott@uwa.edu.au

Heggie TW, Caine DJ (eds): Epidemiology of Injury in Adventure and Extreme Sports.
Med Sport Sci. Basel, Karger, 2012, vol 58, pp 80–97

# The Epidemiology of Injury among Surfers, Kite Surfers and Personal Watercraft Riders: Wind and Waves

Terri J. Pikora[a] · Rebecca Braham[b] · Christina Mills[a]

[a]School of Population Health and [b]School of Sport Science, Exercise and Health at The University of Western Australia, The University of Western Australia, Crawley, W.A., Australia

**Abstract**

The objective of this review was to summarize the epidemiological literature for surfboard riding (surfing), kite surfing and personal watercraft (PWC) riding injuries and describe the incidence and nature of these injuries, common risk factors, and strategies for prevention. The databases searched for relevant publications included Medline, ScienceDirect, ProQuest International, PubMed, Academic Search Premier as well as Google Scholar to identify additional, non-indexed studies. Overall, there was a lack of good quality descriptive studies for these three sports and many of the studies reviewed involved the use of administrative datasets or case-series designs. Among the few studies to provide incidence estimates, there were inconsistencies in how injury was defined, the inclusion criteria, and the reporting of incidence rates, making comparisons within and between the sports difficult. While the reported incidence rates were generally low, head and lower extremity injuries were common across all three sports. Only two studies reported evidence for postulated risk factors. Bigger waves and surfing over rock or reef sea floor increased the risk of injury among competitive surfers, while older age and having more experience increased the risk of significant injuries among recreational surfers. No evaluations of preventative measures were identified. This review demonstrates the need for well-designed epidemiological research, especially studies that focus on the accurate measurement and description of incidence, nature, severity and circumstances of injuries. Once this has occurred, interventions targeted at reducing the incidence of injuries among these sports can be designed, implemented and evaluated.



The adventure and extreme aquatic sporting and recreational pursuits of surfboard riding (surfing), kite surfing and personal watercraft (PWC) riding, also known as jet skis, seadoos and wave runners [1], are popular activities in many countries. While it is difficult to obtain reliable and accurate participant numbers for these sports due to their recreational nature, it is estimated that there are more than 18 million surfers globally [2] and more than 1.45 million PWCs are owned in the USA [3]. Due to the relative newness of kite surfing, participant numbers are more difficult to obtain. It is suggested that these sports are high-risk activities based on the potential for serious injury in addition to acute danger, including the risk of a fatal injury [4–6].

Beginning centuries ago in the South Pacific region, both competitive and recreational surfing has become more popular in recent decades [7, 8]. The basic premise of surfing is to paddle out to an appropriate take-off area, when a suitable wave approaches to paddle with enough speed to 'catch' the wave and to stand up and perform maneuvers on the wave wall until the wave breaks on the shore [8]. This process is repeated many times during each session. The powerful waves and currents of the ocean in combination with a surfboard's sharp fins, rails and nose all present a level of injury risk to a surfer [9]. Recent advances in design and technology have assisted with the development of shorter and lighter boards with improved hydrodynamics, allowing surfers to ride more difficult waves as well as reaching higher speeds [10, 11]. Additional surfing accessories have developed over time including leg ropes, booties, helmets and mouthguards that, when combined with improved wetsuit designs, have meant that surfers are able to surf for longer periods of time and in a range of conditions [12].

A newer development is big wave surfing, although this activity attracts fewer participants compared to the number of surfers. It has been suggested that reasons for this low level of participation is the high level of danger that is posed rather than a lack of accessibility to big waves or due to technological or equipment deficiencies [13]. While injuries are commonplace with a number of highly publicized fatalities, they are rarely reported as surfing injuries, but rather are reported as drowning due to the surfer being held under water by the ocean force [13]. The advent of tow-in surfing, where surfers are towed to larger waves that are not physically possible to paddle to, has further increased the risk of injury amongst big wave surfers [13]. To date, there are no published studies related to injuries among these surfers, therefore this sport is not discussed in this review.

The sport of kite surfing is reasonably new having first been reported to be performed in 1996 [14]. It is unique in that it combines aspects of existing sports including wind surfing, kite flying and water skiing, and involves the use of a small board and a kite which is connected to the surfer by a harness through which wind energy is transferred into speed [5, 15]. The kite is controlled by a handlebar which is connected to the kite by four lines with lengths between 20 and 30 m [5, 15]. Using the vertical lift of the kite, a surfer can perform high jumps even in light surf conditions [5].

While not as old as surfing or as new as kite surfing, PWCs became commercially available in the 1970s with participation rates growing rapidly in recent years [16–19]. This increase in popularity has been attributed to a number of factors including the ease to transport, launch and ride a PWC and the relatively low costs and maintenance compared to other motorized vessels [17]. In addition, more recent models of

PWCs have the capacity to tow a water skier, carry up to three people at once, and are capable of reaching speeds up to 120 km/h [1, 16].

This review summarizes the epidemiological literature on surfing, kite surfing and PWC riding and describes the incidence, nature and causes of injuries, common risk factors and strategies for prevention. Based on this, the objective of the review was to retrieve and report all studies published in English since 1975. Various computer searches were conducted to identify relevant publications using key words: surfing, surfboard riding, wave surfing, kite surfing, jet skiing, water sports, and injury/ies. A range of databases were searched including Medline, ScienceDirect, ProQuest International, PubMed, Academic Search Premier as well as Google Scholar to identify additional studies that were not indexed. Additional papers and reports were identified through the reference lists from sourced review papers, papers and research reports.

There are several limitations in the research reviewed that restrict making comparisons across the studies, including: (1) Many of the studies identified involved the use of a retrospective review of administrative datasets that provide limited ability to explore issues related to injuries in any detail. These datasets include emergency department (ED) presentations [6, 20–22], trauma registries [23–27], hospital admissions [21] and boating accident reports [26, 28, 29]. Other studies explored specific types of injuries (e.g., ocular injuries among surfers [24, 30, 31]; myelopathy among inexperienced surfers [32]), while others collected information from healthcare providers [33–36] or emergency services providing care for injured persons [14–15]. (2) Due to the low number of injuries among these sports, many studies have an insufficient sample size to carry out detailed analysis related to risk factors. (3) There is difficulty in accurately determining the number of persons at risk as most injuries occur during recreational activities where participants are often spread over miles of coastline and any one person may surf or ride in many different localities [33]. In addition, there was no consistent common denominator used in calculating rates across the studies making comparisons difficult. For example hours, days, the number of PWCs in operation are all used. (4) There was wide variability in the definition of injury across the studies. (5) There is frequent use of retrospective, self-report questionnaires among the studies. This methodology is dependent upon memory recollection in relation to both the recall of less serious injuries and time spent pursuing the sport. Many questionnaires had a low response rate (e.g., 37.5% response rate [10]). (6) The use of convenient samples or non-random selection may have resulted in surfers and riders who are seriously injured or who are more concerned with safety and injury prevention to be more often represented in studies. (7) Changes have occurred within these sports over time, for example improvements to surfboard design, improvements to kite surfing safety equipment and more powerful PWC engines, making it difficult to compare results over time. (8) Many of the studies included in this review have been conducted in the USA and Australia, and there may be different practices, issues and safety regulations in other geographical locations.

### Who Is Affected by Injury?

Surfing, kite surfing and PWC riding are often seen as extreme sports with a high risk of injury due to the unpredictability of the ocean and weather conditions that make it attractive to surfers and riders [4, 5]. However, defining injury among these participants is somewhat problematic as many will continue with the activity through an injury and injuries are often seen as inevitable events that are part of participating in their sport [36].

Table 1 provides a comparison of injury rates, collected prospectively and retrospectively, across surfing, kite surfing and PWC riding. As shown, few studies report injury rates for these sports and it is difficult to compare rates among the studies due to differences in exposure measures, definition of an injury or due to small sample sizes. For example, Nathanson et al. [33] conducted a study of injuries requiring medical treatment among competitive surfers worldwide and based the injury rate on hours. In contrast, data collection and reporting methods vary significantly in studies of recreational surfers. Taylor et al. [12] recorded significant acute injuries (those requiring medical attention or time off surfing or work), while an earlier study reported moderate and severe injuries [10] and another utilized hospital admission records for surfboard injuries to estimate rates [11]. Among the studies which reported injuries based on exposure, the rates range from 4.2 overall injuries per 1,000 surfing days [36] to 2.2 significant acute injuries per 1,000 surfing days [7].

Due to the relative newness of the sport, there is a lack of available data for kite surfers. Only two published studies have reported injury rates among recreational kite surfers and these varied from 1.05 per 1,000 h [37] to 7.0 per 1,000 h [5]. These studies are limited in terms of small sample sizes and short time frames as well as differences in study design, thereby limiting comparison between them. There are no published studies addressing injuries among competitive kite surfers.

Only two published studies reported injury rates among recreational jet skiers and these rates were reported as 0.45 per 1,000 h [37] and between 11.8 per 1,000 PWCs in operation during 1990 and 16.2 per 1,000 PWCs in operation in 1995 [6]. Again, these studies are limited in terms of small sample sizes and short time frames as well as differences in study design. Furthermore, the use of the number of PWCs registered to calculate a rate is limited as not all those registered would be used regularly [6]. Similar with kite surfing, there have been no published studies among competitive jet skiers.

Although there is some evidence for injury rates across these sports, much of the data exists at the recreational level with few studies providing evidence based on participation level. In addition, there are consistent methodological limitations in these studies including the definition of injury, study design, sample size and length of data collection. This suggests the need for a more consistent approach across studies, particularly with respect to defining injury and measuring rates, which gives strong grounds for research to continue among these sports.

**Table 1.** Injury rates among surfers, kite surfers and PWC riders

| Activity/study (first author) | Study design | Data collection method | Duration of data collection | Number of injuries | Number of participants | Number of injuries per year/session | Number of injuries per 1,000 h/surfer days |
|---|---|---|---|---|---|---|---|
| Surfers | | | | | | | |
| *Competitive* | | | | | | | |
| Nathanson [2] | R | Q | 6.5 years | 116 (89 during heats) | | competition: 5.7/1,000 heats/surfer significant injuries: 2.9/ 1,000 heats | competition: 13/1,000 h significant injuries: 6.6/1,000 h |
| *Recreational* | | | | | | | |
| Taylor [7] | R | Q | previous 12 months | 168 significant acute 146 chronic health problems | 646 136 | 0.26 injuries/ surfer/year | overall: 2.2/1,000 surfing days |
| Lowdon [10] | R | Q | previous 24 months | 337 | 346 | | moderate/severe: 3.5/1,000 surfing days |
| Allen [11] | R | CR | 56 months | 35 hospitalizations: 24 surfboarding, 11 body surfing | | between 1,969 and 1,975 injuries varied between 1/1,056 and 1/3,683 hospital admissions | severe injury: 1/17,500 surfer days |
| Frisby [36] | R | Q | | 185 | 53 | | overall: 4.2/1,000 surfing days minor: 3.0/1,000 surfing days moderate/major: 1.1/1,000 surfing days |
| Foo [40] | R | Q | | 1,329 | 146 | | |
| Nathanson [33] | R | Q | 4 years | 1,237 acute, 477 chronic injuries | 1348 | | |
| Draper [22] | R | Q | last 2 major injuries last 24 months | 47 | 36 paddlers | | |

**Table 1.** Continued

| Activity/study (first author) | Study design | Data collection method | Duration of data collection | Number of injuries | Number of participants | Number of injuries per year/session | Number of injuries per 1,000 h/surfer days |
|---|---|---|---|---|---|---|---|
| Kite surfers | | | | | | | |
| Pikora [37, 38] | R | Q | previous 12 months | 30 injured at least once in previous year | 57 | | overall: 1.05/1,000 h |
| Nickel [5] | P | Q | 6 months | 124 | 235 | injury risk 2.5 times higher during competition than training | overall: 7.0/1,000 h<br>competition: 16.6/1,000 h<br>exercise/practice: 6.6/1,000 h<br>mild injuries: 5.4/1,000 h<br>medium injuries: 1.4/1,000 h<br>severe injuries: 0.2/1,000 h |
| PWC riders | | | | | | | |
| Pikora [37, 38] | R | Q | previous 12 months | 13 injured at least once in previous year | 47 | | overall: 0.45/ 1,000 h |
| NTSB [29] | R | US Coast Guard PWC accident reports | 6 months | 563 injured, 27 fatal | 500 PWC accidents with injury | | |
| Branche [6] | R | CR<br>ED present-ations<br>PWC-related incident | 6 years | 624 injuries, estimated 32,954 persons injured in US hospital EDs | | | 1990: 11.8/1,000 PWCs in operation; 1991: 8.4/1,000 PWCs; 1992: 10.7/1,000 PWCs; 1993: 9.4/1,000 PWCs; 1994: 11.6/1,000 PWCs; 1995: 16.2/1,000 PWCs |

R = Retrospective; P = prospective; Q = questionnaire; CR = case or chart review.
Where no figures are reported, data were not available within the publication or calculations were not possible from the available data.

### Where Does Injury Occur?

*Anatomical Location*

Highlighting the anatomical location for injuries identifies the body parts that are more likely to be injured which can in turn assist in the development of preventative measures to reduce the number and severity of these injuries. Table 2 shows injury by anatomical location for the three sports. Not all the studies reviewed report injuries by anatomical location and these studies were not included in table.

As shown in table 2, lower extremity injuries were common among surfers with the majority of studies reporting proportions around 40% or higher. The next most frequently injured region was the head followed by the spine and trunk region. These data are difficult to summarize and compare due to the differences in the definition of injury and data collection methods utilized. For example, Taylor et al. [12] surveyed surfers as well as analyzing ED presentation data for surfing injuries and found lower extremity injuries to be more common (45.8%) among survey participants, while head injuries were more common (42.0%) among those attending an ED. Similar results were reported by Nathanson et al. [2] with acute surfing injuries equally common to the head (37.1%) and lower extremities (37.0%), while the head was more common for chronic injuries (36.0%).

Only two published studies reported the anatomical location for kite surfing injuries. As shown in table 2, lower extremity injuries were more common in both these studies with proportion ranging between 38.2 and 53.2% of all injuries [5, 21]. One study described these injuries based on more specific body site and reported that the foot and ankle were more common with 28.2% of all injuries, followed by the skull (13.7%), knee (12.9%) and chest (12.9%) [5]. However, Ashby and Cassell [21] used combined wind and kite surfer data which may not reflect the true nature of injuries among kite surfers.

The vast majority of published studies describing injuries among jet skiers utilized trauma registry data or hospitalization records suggesting that these were serious injuries. Perhaps not surprising, injuries to the head were more common (range 14.8–62.0%) followed by spine and trunk (range 19.5–50.0%) and lower extremities. One study using PWC accident data found that injuries to the lower extremity were more common (34.2%), followed by head (27.8%) and spine and trunk (21.2%) [29]. The use of administrative datasets limits analysis to the information that is routinely collected and none of the studies reported specific body site for injury location.

*Environmental Location*

Environmental factors that have the potential to influence risk for an injury in ocean sports include: waves and currents, wind, impact with stationary objects, impact with floating objects, and impact with other persons [39]. Across all three sports, there is limited information in relation to these factors. In addition, the frequent use of administrative datasets to assess injuries precludes exploring environmental factor

**Table 2.** Anatomical location of injury among surfers, kite surfers and PWC riders

| Activity/study (first author) | Head % | Spine/trunk % | Upper extremity % | Lower extremity % |
|---|---|---|---|---|
| Surfers | | | | |
| *Competitive* | | | | |
| Nathanson [33] | 25.0 | 11.2 | 25.0 | 38.8 |
| *Recreational* | | | | |
| Hay [20] | 41.5 | 14.7 | 22.6 | 18.4 |
| Taylor [12] | | | | |
| *Survey participants | *26.2 | *15.5 | *12.5 | *45.8 |
| **ED visits | **42.0 | **9.7 | **16.1 | **22.8 |
| Foo [40] | 5.9 | 8.7 | 15.7 | 65.9 |
| Nathanson [2] | | | | |
| *Acute injuries | *37.1 | *13.2 | *12.7 | *37.0 |
| **Chronic injuries | **36.0 | **19.0 | **23.0 | **9.0 |
| Draper [22] | | | | |
| *Extrinsic injuries | *11.8 | *11.8 | *23.5 | *49.0 |
| **Intrinsic injuries | | **34.4 | **34.4 | **28.1 |
| Barry [35] | 22.0 | 17.5 | 21.5 | 36.4 |
| Lowdon [10] | 37.0 | 63.0[a] | | |
| Allen [11] | | | | |
| Severe/serious injuries | 27.0 | 51.0 | 9.0 | 6.0 |
| Frisby [36] | | | | |
| Minor injuries | 17.3 | 12.4 | 14.6 | 43.2 |
| Kite surfers | | | | |
| Ashby and Cassell [21] | | | | |
| Wind/kite surfing | 21.8 | 12.4 | 23.5 | 38.2 |
| Nickel [5] | 13.7 | 16.1 | 16.9 | 53.2 |
| PWC riders | | | | |
| Ashby and Cassell [21] | 25.4 | 20.8 | 15.3 | 32.2 |
| Rubin [23] | 55.1 | 19.5 | 17.3[b] | |
| Kim [18] | 33.9 | 40.0 | 3.5 | 22.6 |
| Haan [25] | 62.0 | 50.0 | 21.0[b] | |
| NTSB [29] | 27.8 | 21.2 | 13.3 | 34.2 |
| Jones [28] | 14.8 | | 3.7 | 14.8 |
| Branche [6] | 29.1 | 24.2 | 11.2 | 34.4 |

Where no figures are reported, data were not available within the publication or calculations were not possible from the available data.
[a] This study combined body and extremities into a single category.
[b] This study combined upper and lower extremities into a single category.

information. Furthermore, the reliance of self-report and recollection of environmental factors at the time of an injury may be compromised due to both the retrospective nature of many of the studies as well as the stress associated with an injury.

Few studies have explored the differences in injuries based on whether they occurred in practice or competition. One surfing study compared injuries during surfing competition heats and practice and found 76.7% of injuries occurred during heats [33]. In addition, this study reported an injury rate of 8.7 per 1,000 surfer heats during professional contests compared with 2.7 per 1,000 surfer heats at amateur contests. They suggest that these differences can be explained based on professional contests are more often held in larger surf, over a hard sea floor and are longer in duration [33]. While the numbers were small and three different water sports were combined, Pikora et al. [37] found those who participated in competitions were more likely to have an injury (OR 2.60, 95% CI 1.15–5.85).

Few studies provide information related to environmental factors associated with surfing injuries. Among recreational surfers, common causes of injuries were due to contact with the ocean floor (between 10.0% [36] and 17.9% [2]), hydraulic force of the wave (between 10.0% [36] and 17.0% [2]), and hitting rocks (13.0% [36]). Among kite surfers a high proportion of injuries occurred when on the water (73.0% [37] and 80.0% [5]) followed by between 13.0% [38] and 20.0% [5] occurring when setting up due to a loss of control over the kite. In terms of where injuries occurred, more than half (54%) sustained an injury at a distance >50 m from the beach, with the majority occurring at wind speeds between 11 and 18 knots with flat-water conditions [5]. While it is suggested that most serious injuries sustained during kite surfing are the result of collisions with objects as it is performed near the shore, this was not found among less severe injuries [5, 15]. With increasing popularity for these sports there is the potential for increased risk of injury due to overcrowding in popular locations. Only one study has explored the issue of numbers in the water at the time of injury. This study reported that at the time of injury there was an average of 14 other surfers in the water [2]. However, this average number increased to 19 when another's surf board caused the injury [2].

## When Does Injury Occur?

### *Injury Onset*

There is limited information related to injury onset among surfing in the studies reviewed and none for the other two sports. Two studies have reported both acute and chronic injuries among surfers. Among recreational surfers, 37.0% reported a chronic injury with overuse syndromes (including shoulder, back, neck and knee strain) being most common [2]. Other chronic conditions found were related to prolonged exposure to sun and seawater with the most common being exostosis of the ear (or surfer's ear) [2]. Similar results were found by Taylor et al. [12] with 21.1%

of respondents in their survey reporting a chronic condition that was attributed to surfing generally not to an acute injury. Most common were ear problems (45.9%) followed by musculoskeletal problems (38.4%) and general muscle and joint pain or stiffness (9.6%) [12].

*Chronometry*
Limited information is available about the chronometry of injuries among surfers, kite surfers and PWC riders in the studies reviewed. Only one study reported that 77% of all surfing injuries occurred during the summer months [20]. Many of the studies included in this review used administrative datasets to identify injuries or have used short timeframes thereby limiting the ability to determine timing of when the injury occurred. It would be useful to determine when injuries occur, either in terms of the season, time of the day, or time into practice, to assist in identifying whether more injuries occur if and when fatigue is an issue as well as environmental conditions.

### What Is the Outcome?

*Injury Type*
Due to differences in defining and classifying injury types across the studies, difficulties arise when making comparisons. In addition, there are vast differences when utilizing self-report results compared with those collected from administrative datasets. Table 3 shows the comparison across the type of injury for each of the three sports. The most common type of injury among surfers were lacerations (15.5–63.0%) followed by sprains and strains (2.0–38.8%). Among those with serious injuries, fractures were found to be prevalent (77.3%), while another found abrasions to be more common (41.1%). Injuries involving marine animals were rarely reported in these papers.

As shown in table 3, only two studies reported the type of injury among kite surfers. Ashby and Cassell [21] reported more fractures (37.6%) than Nickel et al. [5] possibly due to the different data collection methods used, while Nickel et al. reported contusions to be more common (33.8%). As the former study reviewed more serious injuries among both windsurfers and kite surfers based on hospitalizations and ED presentations [21] while the later conducted a prospective study among kite surfers [5], it is difficult to identify common injuries for kite surfing based on the results of these two studies.

The injury type data presented among PWC riders were based on hospitalizations, ED presentations and trauma registries reflecting that these were more serious injuries. As shown in table 3, lacerations were more common among PWC riders (between 11.0 and 78.0%) followed by fractures (between 12.4 and 68.0%) and contusions (between 7.0 and 25.4%).

**Table 3.** Type of injury in surfers, kite surfers and PWC riders

| Activity/ study | Abrasion % | Concussion % | Contusion % | Dislocation % | Fracture % | Laceration % | Sprain/ strain % | Strain % | Other % |
|---|---|---|---|---|---|---|---|---|---|
| Surfers | | | | | | | | | |
| *Competitive* | | | | | | | | | |
| Nathanson [33] | 5.2 | | 8.6 | | 8.6[a] | 30.2 | 38.8 | | 7.8 |
| *Recreational* | | | | | | | | | |
| Hay [20] | | | | | | | | | |
| *Minor/moderate injuries | | | | *12.6 | *13.7 | | | | |
| **Serious injuries | | | *13.7 | **9.1 | **77.3 | *36.4 | *21.0 | | **13.6 |
| Taylor [12] | | | | | | | | | |
| *Survey participants | | | | *10.7 | *8.9 | *46.4 | *28.6 | | *5.4 |
| **ED visits | | | | **2.2 | **14.2 | **47.2 | **12.4 | | **24.0 |
| Foo [40] | | | 37.0 | 1.4 | 3.8 | 54.7 | 3.1 | | 0.0 |
| Nathanson [2] | | 5.9 | 12.6 | | 8.1 | 42.3 | 12.0 | | 19.1 |
| Grenfell [34] | | | 5.0 | 1.0 | 4.0 | 63.0 | 10.0 | | 15.0 |
| Draper [22] | | | | | 3.9 | 47.1 | 2.0 | | 47.0 |
| Barry [35] | 41.4 | | | | 2.9 | 15.5 | 3.2 | | 36.1 |
| Lowdon [10] | | | 38.0 | | 15.0 | 41.0 | 35.0[b] | | |
| Frisby [36] | 10.1 | 4.2 | 29.2 | 0.5 | 0.5 | 19.1 | 9.6 | 7.5 | 19.1 |
| Kite surfers | | | | | | | | | |
| Ashby and Cassell Wind/ kite surfing | | 5.9 | 7.1 | | 37.6 | 14.1 | 21.2[c] | | 9.4 |
| Nickel [5] | 27.4 | | 33.8 | | 3.2 | 16.9 | 9.7 | 1.6 | 7.3 |
| PWC riders | | | | | | | | | |
| Ashby and Cassell [21] | 7.0 | 3.9 | 7.0 | | 27.8 | 16.7 | 15.0[c] | | 21.0 |
| White [41] | | 13.0 | | | 28.0 | 78.0[d] | | | |
| Shatz [27] | | | | | 68.0 | | | | |
| Jones [28] | 4.0 | | | | 19.0 | 11.0 | 4.0 | | 13.0 |
| Branche [6] | | | 25.4 | | 12.4 | 30.8 | 18.7 | | 12.7 |
| Hammam [26] | | | | | 26.0 | 57.0 | | | |

Where no figures are reported, data were not available within the publication or calculations were not possible from the available data.
[a] This study combined fractures and dislocations into a single category.
[b] This study combined sprains and strains into a single category.
[c] This study combined dislocations, sprains and strains into a single category.
[d] This study combined lacerations and contusions into a single category.

*Injury Severity*

Few studies have reported injury severity data among surfers, kite surfers and PWC riders. However, among those to have done so, there were differences in the definition of severity and how these data were presented. Typically, among all three water sports, severity has been defined by level of care required to treat the injury and by the time lost due to an injury, although these definitions vary between studies. Measures of severity have been described among the surfing injury studies based on the level of care required to treat an injury, although there were differences in the presentation of this information. Many surfing injuries are seen as minor with a range between 42% minor cuts [35], 90% minor/moderate [20], 72.4% minor [36], 33% minor [2], and 9.5% treatment required from medical doctor [40]. Another measure of severity is time off from surfing. One study reported that among those who were injured, 43.4% lost 1–3 and 39.6% lost 4–14 days of surfing [10]. Due to these inconsistencies, it is difficult to draw conclusions related to the level of injury severity.

Only two studies describe the severity of kite surfing injuries. Nickel et al. [5] reported 77% of all injuries were mild (5.4/1,000 kite surfing hours); 19% medium (1.4/1,000 h) with the remaining 3% severe (0.2/1,000 h) [5]. In this study mild injuries were defined as the incapacity to train or compete on a normal basis, medium as absence from kite surfing for more than 1 day, and severe injuries as absence from kite surfing for more than 6 weeks. In contrast, Pikora et al. [38] describe injuries based on level of treatment required, with 44.1% of injuries required first aid, 20.6% treatment from a rehabilitation specialist (e.g. physiotherapist), 10.3% ED visit, 7.4% treatment from a general practitioner and 2.9% a hospital admission. It is difficult to draw conclusions on injury severity based on these two studies although it would appear that most self-reported injuries are minor.

The vast majority of studies among PWC riders were based on administrative datasets reflecting the more serious nature of these injuries and with higher numbers of fatalities than the other two sports. Based on US Coast Guard data, the majority of injuries were minor (61.4%) with 25.1% considered moderate and 8.1% as serious injuries [29]. Using an injury severity rating based on level of treatment required, survey respondents reported that 25.8% of injuries required first aid, 12.9% an ED visit, 12.9% treatment from a general practitioner, 9.7% treatment from a rehabilitation specialist (e.g. physiotherapist) and 3.2% a hospital admission [38]. One study analyzed trauma registry data for pediatric patients aged between 5 and 19 years and found that 42.4% had a functional disability and that 9.1% of these had a long-term disability [23]. Another study reported the length of stay for hospital admission was 4.4 ± 3.5 days and intensive care length of stay of 3.6 ±4.8 days for injured PWC riders [41].

*Clinical Outcome*

There is limited information related to the clinical outcomes of injury among surfers presented in the studies reviewed with no clinical outcomes reported among kite surfers and PWC riders. Taylor et al. [12] reported that 3.1% of surfers reported long-term effects as a result of an acute injury including unstable or painful or stiff joints, chronic skin ulcers, and loss of teeth. The vast majority of PWC rider studies have sourced information related to injuries and fatalities from administrative datasets. As a result, these injuries are often more serious and report a higher number of fatalities than when information is collected at the community level and in the field rather than at the place of treatment.

*Economic Cost*

There was limited economic cost information related to injury among surfers presented in the studies reviewed with no data available for either kite surfers or PWC riders. Typically, this information is provided either in terms of time off work or surfing (e.g., time off work or surfing [12], disabled for more than one day [2]), the level of disability [23] or the number of days spent in hospital [41] providing limited opportunity to compare across the studies. Two surfing studies provide information related to the number of days the injury resulted in time off work or surfing while another used 'disabled for more than one day'. The proportion of surfers with an injury that required days off or were disabled ranged between 26% for significant injuries (disabled for more than one day [2]) and 67.3% with a mean of 4.3 ± 5.5 weeks and range of 2 days to 50 weeks (days off work or surfing [12]). Unfortunately, across all three sports, there is no data available on the cost of treatment as a result of injury.

## What Are the Risk Factors?

An in-depth knowledge of injury risk factors is important to inform and guide effective injury prevention, intervention and rehabilitation programs. However, there is a lack of analytical studies related to risk factors among these sports available in the published literature. Only one study among competitive surfers identified risk factors for surfing-related injuries during surfing heats [33]. In this study, the adjusted risk for injury was 2.4 (95% CI 1.5–3.9) times greater when surfing in waves overhead or bigger compared with waves less than overhead and 2.6 (95% CI 1.3–5.2) times greater when surfing over a rock or reef bottom compared to a sandy bottom [33]. Another study among recreational surfers found that, when compared to minor injuries, the risk for a significant injury was almost double among surfers aged 40 years or more compared with those aged 20 years or less (OR 1.9, 95% CI 1.1–3.4) and higher among those who rated their level of ability as advanced or expert and professional compared to novice or intermediate (OR 1.6, 95% CI 1.1–2.3; OR 1.9, 95% CI 1.1–3.4 respectively) [2]. In addition, the risk for significant injury in waves overhead or higher was twice that of smaller waves (OR 2.0, 95% CI 1.3–3.3) [2]. An earlier study by Lowdon et al. [10] reported a correlation between increased surfing competence and the incidence of head lacerations ($r = 0.18$; $p < 0.001$), skull fractures

($r = 0.13$; $p < 0.001$) and other skeletal fractures ($r = 0.09$; $p < 0.05$). One explanation proffered was that the more competent a surfer became, the more often they choose more difficult surf and over shallow reefs while a beginner will generally surf smaller breaks [10].

### What Are the Inciting Events?

There is limited information related to the inciting events leading to an injury presented in the studies reviewed. Surfing injuries as a result of impact with a surfboard was reported for a proportion of injuries among both recreational (between 45.2% [7] and 67.0% [2]) and competitive surfers (29.0% [33]), with this impact being from their own board between 37.0% [36] and 82.0% [2] of the time. One recreational and one competitive surfing injury study determined when the injury occurred related to the maneuver attempted at the time [2, 33]. Among recreational surfers more acute injuries were sustained when riding a wave (62.0%), with 16.0% of these following an unsuccessful takeoff, 16% following a turning maneuver and 10.0% when riding a tube [2]. Similarly, competitive surfers were more likely to be injured due to an unsuccessful takeoff (25.0%), 20.0% followed a turning maneuver and 16.0% when tube riding [33].

When kite surfers were asked about what caused the injury, 44.0% reported that it was due to technical mistake with 30.6% reporting to have mislanded a jump [5]. Other common reasons for injury included landing awkwardly (47.0%), an injury due to equipment (23.0%), and attempting something beyond control/skill level (23.0%) [38]. In addition, 24.0% of injuries occurred due to an overestimated of their expertise and 15.0% due to misinterpretation of the weather conditions [5].

PWC rider injuries are often the result of a collision, although the majority of the studies in this review were based on serious injuries sourced from administrative datasets. Collisions are reported to be the most common cause of injuries among PWC riders with many of these the result of colliding with another PWC or with a fixed or stationary object [21, 23, 25–26, 28–29, 41]. There is a lack of consistency among the studies both in the provision of data related to collisions and the information provided in relation to what the rider collided with. This may be due to the use of administrative data that limits exploring these issues in more detail. In contrast, a more recent survey reported a higher proportion of injuries were the result of landing awkwardly (77.0%) and only 15.0% as a result of a collision [38].

The risk of injury may be increased through the use of alcohol and illicit drug due to slower reaction times, impaired judgment and reduced inhibitions [39]. Few studies, and no kite surfing studies, report alcohol and illicit drugs as a contributing factor for injuries among these sports and of those that did, these rates were low. While an optional question, 1% of recreational surfers reported being under the influence of drugs or alcohol [2]. Among PWC riders, the involvement of alcohol ranged between

5.0% [1, 27, 29] and 8.3% [25] of injuries. However, these results may reflect the use self-report method of data collection where participants may underreport negative behaviors, including alcohol and drug use, and with the use of administrative datasets that restricts exploring these issues in more detail.

### Injury Prevention

More information related to injury prevention is required, as this was found to be inadequate in the studies reviewed. In addition, there are no evaluations of interventions and equipment modifications reported to prevent injuries among these sports. It has been suggested that there has been a limited focus upon prevention strategies among any ocean-related sports injuries in relation to the dangers of natural aquatic environments, including those related to currents, waves and the ocean floor, as well as targeting transient groups [39]. To date, there have been no published evaluations of injury prevention interventions or equipment modifications among either surfers or PWC riders, although there are several areas for prevention that are postulated to reduce injury in the literature including protective headgear and design improvements [19, 42, 43]. While the numbers were small and three different water sports were combined, Pikora et al. [37] found that compared with those who used fewer items of protective equipment, those who used more items of protective equipment were less likely to be injured in the previous 12 months (OR 0.39, 95% CI 0.16–0.92 for between 3 and 5 items and OR 0.60, 95% CI 0.22–1.59 for more than 6 items).

Few studies have explored the use of equipment among kite surfers to prevent or reduce the severity of injuries. One study reported that only 21% of kite surfers used any protective devices, with 7% wearing a helmet and 18% using a quick-release system that enables the surfer to release the kite when they lose control [5]. The injury rate among those who did use a quick-release system was lower than those who did not (4.8/1,000 h compared with 7.6/1,000 h) although this was not statistically significant [5].

### Further Research

This review summarized the existing injury literature about the aquatic sporting and recreational pursuits of surfing, kite surfing and PWC riding. Overall, it is evident that injuries are an important issue for these extreme aquatic sports. Using this information, there are several recommendations for future research:

(1) Research definitions of 'injury' as well as exposure rate measures and economic costs are often inconsistent and vary considerably across studies. Therefore, it is necessary to elucidate key definitions and to create consistent measures so that comparative population-based studies can be conducted across different geographical locations as well as across the different sports.

(2) It remains important to accurately determine exposure rates for these sports for the calculation of injury rates which allows comparison across different geographical locations as well as across different sports.

(3) In order to overcome the existing reliance on administrative data, future research should look to new and innovative ways to recruit and collect data (e.g. via online community surveys) and identify improved methods of injury surveillance to measure the full scope of injuries. The transient and locational nature of these sports, together with the high number of recreational participants, makes it imperative to utilize recruitment strategies that cover a wide range of locations.

(4) Body regions that are common sites for serious injuries appear to be head and spine/trunk with lacerations, fractures and musculoskeletal injuries prevalent. However, the accuracy of these data may be questionable given the variety of data collection methods used along with small participant numbers and short time frames. To improve reliability, validity and precision, larger, longitudinal studies are recommended to allow the measurement of injuries over time and assess the impact of injuries and other chronic health conditions as people age.

(5) Few studies have been conducted into injuries based on whether they occur among competitive or recreational participants. It remains important to determine any differences through recruiting across all levels of participation in large enough numbers to determine the focus for preventative strategies.

(6) There is a lack of analytical studies that provide the ability to either identify or quantify the level of risk for the factors that may influence injury (e.g. environmental conditions, overcrowding, the role of alcohol and drugs). It remains essential to identify both target groups and preventive strategies. In addition, no evaluation studies currently exist of preventive measures. Studies are needed to determine the effects of injury prevention programs and other interventions upon the incidence and reduction in the severity of injuries.

(7) Further research is also required to assess the rehabilitation outcomes and the incidence of residual disabilities among severely injured cases as well as the financial costs related to injuries.

(8) With new sports evolving and pushing the boundaries, it will be important to monitor injuries and to assess preventative measures among these sports. Examples of these include tow-in surfing and big wave surfing.

## References


1 Latch R, Fiser DH: The increasing threat of personal watercraft injuries. Clin Pediatr 2004;43:309–311.

2 Nathanson A, Haynes P, Galanis D: Surfing injuries. Am J Emerg Med 2002;20:155–160.

3 Personal Watercraft Industry Association: The history, evolution and profile of personal watercraft: a report by the Personal Watercraft Industry Association, Washington 2006. Retrieved from http://www.pwia.org/UserFiles/File/History-PWC.pdf

4 Diehm R, Armatas C: Surfing: an avenue for socially acceptable risk-taking, satisfying needs for sensation seeking and experience seeking. Pers Individ Dif 2004;36:663–677.
5 Nickel C, Zernial O, Musahl V, Hansen U, Zantop T, Petersen W: A prospective study of kite-surfing injuries. Am J Sports Med 2004;32:921–927.
6 Branche C, Conn J, Annest J: Personal watercraft-related injuries. JAMA 1997;278:663–665.
7 Taylor KS, Zoltan TB, Achar SA: Medical illnesses and injuries encountered during surfing. Curr Sports Med Rep 2006;5:262–267.
8 Mendez-Villanueva A, Bishop D: Physiological aspects of surfboard riding performance. Sports Med 2005;35:55–70.
9 Sunshine S: Surfing injuries. Curr Sports Med Rep 2003;2:136–141.
10 Lowdon BJ, Pateman NA, Pitman AJ: Surfboard-riding injuries. Med J Aust 1983;2:613–616.
11 Allen RH, Eiseman B, Straehley CJ, Orloff BG: Surfing injuries at Waikiki. JAMA 1977;237:668–670.
12 Taylor DM, Bennett D, Carter M, Garewal D, Finch C: Acute injury and chronic disability resulting from surfboard riding. J Sci Med Sport 2004;7:429–437.
13 Olivier S: Moral dilemmas of participation in dangerous leisure activities. Leisure Stud 2006;25:95–109.
14 Exadaktylos AK, Sclabas GM, Blake I, Swemmer K, McCormick G, Erasmus P: The kick with the kite: an analysis of kite surfing related offshore rescue missions in Cape Town, South Africa. Br J Sports Med 2005;39:e26.
15 Spanjersberg WR, Schipper IB: Kitesurfing: when fun turns to trauma – the dangers of a new extreme sport. J Trauma 2007;63:E76–E80.
16 Cassell E, Congiu M: Review of the literature on the epidemiology and prevention of unintentional submersion and non-submersion injury in recreational boating. Melbourne, Marine Safety Victoria, 2007. Retrieved from http://www.marinesafety.vic.gov.au/doi/doielect.nsf/2a6bd98dee287482ca256915001cff0c/2cc27bcc69173ee7ca2572d40020a451/$FILE/Submersion%20injury%20-%20Recreational%20Boat.pdf
17 Whitfield R, Roche R: UK personal watercraft management: a user perspective. Marine Policy 2007;31:564–572.
18 Kim CW, Smith JM, Lee A, Hoyt DB, Kennedy F, Newton PO, Meyer RS: Personal watercraft injuries: 62 patients admitted to the San Diego County trauma services. J Orthop Trauma 2003;17:571–573.
19 Burger J, Leonard J: Conflict resolution in coastal waters: the case of personal watercraft. Marine Policy 2000;24:61–67.
20 Hay CSM, Barton S, Sulkin T: Recreational surfing injuries in Cornwall, United Kingdom. Wilderness Environ Med 2009;20:335–338.
21 Ashby K, Cassell E: Marine Safety in Victoria: Report to Marine Safety Victoria. Melbourne, Monash University Accident Research Centre, 2009. Retrieved from http://www.marinesafety.vic.gov.au/DOI/DOIElect.nsf/$UNIDS+for+Web+Display/FA5B89EC4D126834CA25764200101230/$FILE/4096%20MSV%205%20Year%20Report%20WEB.pdf
22 Draper JA, Pyne DB, Thompson KM, Fricker PA: Injury occurrence in surf board and surf ski paddlers. Aust J Sci Med Sport 1987;19:20–22.
23 Rubin LE, Stein PB, DiScala C, Grottkau BE: Pediatric trauma caused by personal watercraft: a ten-year retrospective. J Pediatr Surg 2003;38:1525–1529.
24 Kim JW, McDonald HR, Rubsamen PE, Luttrull JK, Drouilhet JH, Frambach DA, Boyer DS, Lambrou FH, Hendrick A, Weis JN, Engstrom RE, Ing M: Surfing-related ocular injuries. Retina 1998;18:424–429.
25 Haan J, Kramer M, Scalea T: Pattern of injury from personal watercraft. Am Surg 2002;68:624–627.
26 Hamman B, Miller F, Fallat M, Richardson JD: Injuries resulting from motorized personal watercraft. J Pediatr Surg 2003;28:920–922.
27 Shatz D, Kirton O, McKenney M, Ginzburg E, Byers PM, Augenstein JS, Sleeman D, Auguila Z: Personal watercraft crash injuries: an emerging problem. J Trauma 1998;44:198–201.
28 Jones CS: Children and personal watercraft: injury characteristics and potential countermeasures. Inj Prev 1998;4:61–62.
29 National Transportation Safety Board: Safety study: personal watercraft safety. Springfield, Virginia, National Transportation Safety Board, 1998. Retrieved from http://www.ridetechnology.com/NTSBPWCSafetyStudy.pdf
30 Zoumalan CI, Blumenkranz MS, McCulley TJ, Moshfeghi DM: Severe surfing-related ocular injuries: the Stanford Northern Californian experience. Br J Sports Med 2008;42:855–857.
31 Lawless M, Pountney R, Porter W, Simpson M: Surfboard-related ocular injuries. Aust NZ J Ophthalmol 1986;14:55–57.
32 Thompson TP, Pearce J, Chang G, Madamba J: Surfer's myelopathy. Spine 2004;16:E353–E356.

33 Nathanson A, Bird S, Dao L, Tam-Sing K: Competitive surfing injuries: a prospective study of surfing-related injuries among contest surfers. Am J Emerg Med 2007;35:113–117.
34 Grenfell RD: Beach-related injuries (letter). Med J Aust 1996;166:390.
35 Barry SW, Kleinig BJ, Brophy T: Surfing injuries. Aust J Sports Med 1982;14:49–51.
36 Frisby R: Surfing injuries in Otago and Southland, New Zealand. Southern Institute of Technology (no date). Retrieved from http://blackmagic.com/ses/surfpapers/NZsurfinjury.pdf
37 Pikora TJ, Braham R, Hill C, Mills C: Wet and wild: results from a pilot study assessing injuries among recreational water users in Western Australia. Int J Inj Contr Saf Promot 2011;18:119–126.
38 Pikora TJ, Hill C, Braham R, Mills C: Wet and wild: assessing injuries among recreational water users in Western Australia. Perth, Australia. School of Population Health, University of Western Australia, 2010.
39 Hartung GH, Goebert DA: Ocean sports; in Caine DJ, Caine CG, Lindner KJ (eds): Epidemiology of Sports Injuries. Champaign/Ill, Human Kinetics, 1996, pp 284–300.
40 Foo P, Nicholls B: Surfing injuries in recreational surfers. Department of Human Development, School of Health Sciences, Victoria University of Technology, 2004. Retrieved from http://eptest.vu.edu.au/712/1/Foo_et_al_2004.pdf
41 White MW, Cheatham ML: The underestimated impact of personal watercraft injuries. Am Surg 1999;65:865–869.
42 Taylor DM, Bennett D, Carter M, Garewal D, Finch C: Perceptions of surfboard riders regarding the need for protective headgear. Wilderness Environ Med 2005;16:75–80.
43 Chalmers DJ, Morrison L: Epidemiology of non-submersion injuries in aquatic sporting and recreational activities. Sports Med 2003;33:745–770.



Terri J. Pikora, MPH, PhD
School of Population Health at The University of Western Australia
M431, The University of Western Australia
35 Stirling Highway, Crawley, WA 6009 (Australia)
Tel. +61 8 0418883985, E-Mail terri.pikora@uwa.edu.au

Heggie TW, Caine DJ (eds): Epidemiology of Injury in Adventure and Extreme Sports.
Med Sport Sci. Basel, Karger, 2012, vol 58, pp 98–111

# The Epidemiology of Injury in Canoeing, Kayaking and Rafting

Richard C. Franklin[a,c] · Peter A. Leggat[a,b]

[a]World Safety Organisation Collaborating Centre for Injury Prevention and Safety Promotion and Anton Breinl Centre for Public Health & Tropical Medicine, School of Public Health, Tropical Medicine and Rehabilitation Sciences, James Cook University, Townsville, Qld., Australia; [b]School of Public Health, University of Witwatersrand, Johannesburg, South Africa, and [c]Royal Life Saving Society, Broadway, N.S.W., Australia

**Abstract**

The aquatic environment is a complex mix of waterways with varying uses and hazards. It is the intersection of the use of the water and the hazards which provides enjoyment to those who use them as well as risk to a person's health. Canoeing, kayaking and rafting have and continue to be popular recreation sports in aquatic environments. This chapter explores participation in, risks associated with and prevention strategies for keeping canoeists, kayakers and rafters safe and healthy. There is a dearth of good quality descriptive studies exploring these issues, particularly around the risks involved and the effectiveness of proposed prevention strategies. According to Outdoor Foundation, there are 23.9 million people in the USA who undertake paddling activities per annum, with canoeing (10.1 million) being the most popular activity followed by recreational kayaking (6.2 million). There were 141 deaths of canoeists (89) and kayakers (52) identified by the US Coast Guard in their recreational boating statistics data for 2009. The crude rate of death per 100,000 participants for canoeing ranges between 0.72 and 0.92 and for kayaking between 0.37 and 0.41 per annum. Although death is the most severe consequence of a misadventure while paddling, there are a range of other hazards faced such as hitting objects, waterborne diseases, hypothermia from unintended submersion, blisters, muscle strain, cuts and abrasions. There are a range of prevention strategies which have been proposed and provided in this chapter. However, there is very little evidence of their effectiveness. Further research is required in understanding the risk associated with paddling activities, the effectiveness of prevention strategies and how these strategies might be delivered.



The use of the aquatic environment for sport and recreation is not new with boating regattas being held in the 1800s and the now famous 'The Boat Race' between Oxford University and Cambridge University started in 1829 and continues to this day. What has changed over the ensuing years is the type and variety of aquatic activity, which can be undertaken, with some people embracing recreational pursuits in conditions that test them to their limits.

Added to this is the competition for the tourism dollar, where more and varied activities are being delivered to attract and increase the number of people who visit a country, region, or town. For those areas, which have access to aquatic locations, these are being used for a range of adventure sports or to attract people interested in knowing more about the natural environment. Unfortunately, this interaction brings with it a range of hazards, although with proper preparation the risk of the hazards causing major injuries, illness or death can be minimized. However, those people who are seeking adventure activities are often required to visit remote, rural areas, where medical help is difficult to obtain [1] and where standard travel insurance coverage may not extend [2].

A risk assessment and risk management approach are essential in ensuring safety when undertaking any activity. Most people who undertake an activity do not do so with the intent to end up severely injured or dead. For those individuals with little or no experience, they are reliant on those teaching them or taking them on the activity to ensure their safety. In order to conduct a review of the epidemiological data associated with canoeing, kayaking, and rafting, a search for relevant publications was conducted using PubMed, Medline, Science Direct, Google Scholar, ProQuest International, and Academic Search Premier. While there is a dearth of good quality descriptive studies exploring these issues, drowning was identified as the major risk faced when in, on, or around water. In fact, each year between 400,000 and 1.2 million people drown globally [3, 4]. The majority of those who drown do so close to home and a good number of those who drown while undertaking recreational activities are from Western countries. For people travelling the risk of drowning is not insubstantial, an Australian study found that while three quarters (73%) of the deaths to overseas visitors was natural causes, 5% of people drowned while on their vacation to Australia [5]. Drowning was a major cause of preventable death in a number of similar studies of travellers around the world.

### *Canoeing, Kayaking and Rafting*

For the purposes of this chapter, we have grouped those activities which require padding, i.e. those activities which require a person to use a paddle to maneuver a vessel through the water. Mainly this refers to canoeing, kayaking and rafting. These activities primarily involve the use of the arms and the need for a level of aerobic fitness [6]. While there are differences between the vessels, traditionally a kayak was a closed boat where an individual's legs are under cover and a canoe was an open boat. There are now a range of different vessels such as a sea kayak where a person kneels or stands to paddle.

In 2009, there were 23.9 million people in the USA who participated in paddling activities (table 1) [7]. Canoeists tend to be male (60%), Caucasian (86%), and aged 25+ years (25–44, 34%; 45+, 28%) with about a half (49%) earning over USD 75,000 per annum. Rafters are also predominately male (60%), Caucasian (81%), and aged 25+ years (25–44, 40%; 45+, 25%), with half (50%) earning over USD 75,000 per annum. Kayakers

**Table 1.** Number of participants (millions) in the USA, 2006–2009 (source: Outdoor Foundation, 2010)

| | 2006 | 2007 | 2008 | 2009 |
|---|---|---|---|---|
| Canoeing | 9.2 | 9.8 | 9.9 | 10.1 |
| Rafting | 3.6 | 4.6 | 4.7 | 4.3 |
| Kayaking (recreational) | 4.1 | 5.1 | 6.2 | 6.2 |
| Kayaking (sea/touring) | 1.1 | 1.5 | 1.8 | 1.8 |
| Kayaking (white water) | 0.8 | 1.2 | 1.2 | 1.4 |

were also predominately male (56%), Caucasian (82%), and aged 25+ years (25–44, 36%; 45+, 30%), with just over half (57%) earning over USD 75,000 per annum [8].

In a 2009 survey investigating what motivates people to participate in outdoor activities such as canoeing, kayaking, and rafting, the Outdoor Industry Association and Outdoor Foundation identified the six most common reasons as: it is relaxing, it is a great way to get exercise, it is fun, I enjoy discovery and exploration, I want to be healthy, and I get away from my usual routine. The order of these changed depending on the activity, e.g. it is relaxing was the top reason for kayakers and rafters, whereas it is fun was the top reason for canoeists. It is also interesting to note that friends, parents and other relatives (such as brother and sister) are significant in a person's decision to participate in outdoor activities [8].

### Who Is Affected by Injury?

Canoeing, kayaking and rafting are undertaken by a wide variety of people and injury can occur to any person who participates in these activities. For example, in a survey of white-water rafting guides, 77.4% of the respondents reported back pain while guiding [9]. In a study of sea kayaking incidents in New Zealand, they occurred all year to people from a range of ages. However, males (85%) were more likely than female (10%) to be involved in an incident [10].

Each year the US Coast Guard compiles the number of deaths due to recreational boating fatalities in the USA. The number of deaths overall for canoeing and kayaking have been increasing over the years with 141 recorded deaths in 2010. However, there was a slight decrease in the number of canoeing deaths in 2010 (table 2) [11–15]. While these reports also provide injury counts, the number of injuries is lower than the number of deaths. As such, the authors have considered this information to be unreliable.

In 2010, there were 6 people under the age of 12 who died (4 while canoeing and 2 while kayaking), with the most common age group being the 20- to 29-year group with 40 deaths followed by the 50- to 59-year age group with 29 deaths (fig. 1) [15].

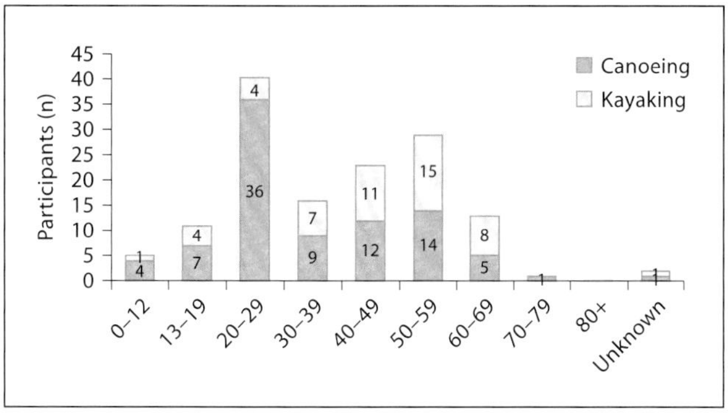


**Fig. 1.** Age groupings of canoe and kayaking participants, 2010.

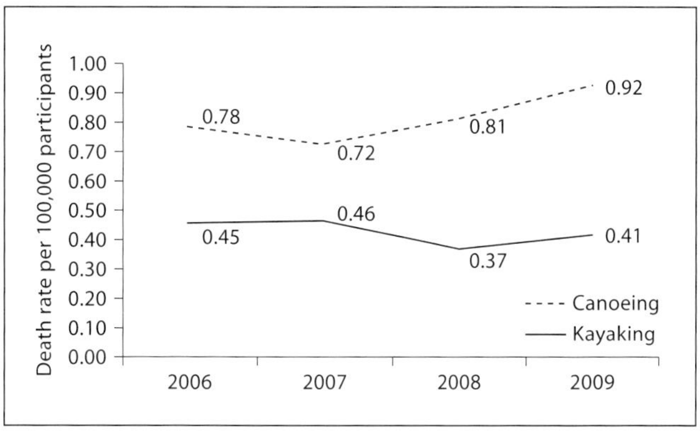


**Fig. 2.** Crude rate of death by participation for canoeing and kayaking, 2006–2009.

**Table 2.** Deaths while participating in canoeing or kayaking activities, 2006–2009 (source: US Coast Guard Recreational Boating Statistics, 2006–2010)

| Deaths | 2006 | 2007 | 2008 | 2009 | 2010 |
|---|---|---|---|---|---|
| Canoeing | 72 | 71 | 80 | 93 | 89 |
| Kayaking | 27 | 36 | 34 | 39 | 52 |
| Total | 99 | 107 | 114 | 132 | 141 |

The crude rate of death per 100,000 participants ranged from 0.72 to 0.92 for canoe-related deaths and from 0.37 to 0.41 for kayak-related deaths (fig. 2). Common contributing factors for canoe deaths and injuries recorded by the US Coast Guard included alcohol use (22; 18%), hazardous waters (22; 18%), improper loading (15; 12.5%), operator inexperience (15; 12.5%) and weather (10; 8%). For kayak-related deaths the most common contributing factor identified by the US Coast Guard was hazardous waters (41; 45%) [15]. The most common result of the contributing factors was capsizing for both canoe- (78; 65%) and kayak-related (48; 52%) deaths and injuries [15].

While death is one possible outcome from undertaking paddling activities, there are a range of other injuries which can and do occur. A study by Kameyama et al. [19] of the Japan Canoe Association found that more than half (54.9%) of the 417 study respondents reported some physical problem during paddling. In a survey of white-water rafting guides, three quarters (77.4%) report some back pain [9]. Thus it could be concluded that all people who undertake any of the paddling activities are at risk.

## Where Does the Injury Occur?

Although death is the most severe consequence of a misadventure while kayaking or rafting, these are reasonably rare events with a fatality rate per million participant days of 2.2–8.7 for kayaking [16] and 4.5–8.7 for rafting [16, 17]. There are a range of both anatomical and geographical locations where the injuries occur. However, while knowing information about these provides greater detail in which to help develop injury prevention measures, more information is required about the circumstances leading to either injury or death for people who undertake canoeing, kayaking or rafting activities.

### *Anatomical Locations*

According to Whisman and Hollenhorst [18], the body areas more commonly injured were the face (33%) (including the eye, mouth, nose and teeth), knee (15%), arm/wrist/hand (11.6%), and other parts of the leg/hip/foot (11%). This was also supported by a study from Japan where they found that respondents experienced lumbago (22.5%), shoulder pain (20.9%), wrist pain (10.8%) and elbow pain (3.8%) [19]. For kayakers in the sea environment, injury or medical conditions which have been found to commonly occur include: sprains and pulled muscles (19.7%), cuts and abrasions (19%), painful or stiff back (12.1%), sunburn (11.7%) blisters (11.0%), and painful joints and tendons (11.0%). It should also be noted that concussion hypothermia, near-drowning, and dislocation have also been found to occur. While all anatomical locations have been found to be injured the most common for kayakers in the sea environment include: back (17.9%), hand (12.7%), shoulder (11.6%), and head (10.4%) [20].

Injuries do not only occur to recreational participants. For example, a study of athletes who participated in the 1996 Olympic trials for white-water paddling found that traumatic injuries were the most common type of injury and the torso and back were the most frequent sites with strain being the most common occurrence. Other anatomical locations injured included the shoulder (of which 15% were considered to be severe) [21].

Injuries have also been found to occur to the back, this was particularly highlighted in a study of white-water rafting guides where 77.4% of guides reported back pain an 20.8% had back pain lasting more than a week. It should also be noted that the back pain may not only be related to the activity but also to the moving of the raft [9]. Hyperthermia was also found to be an issue, along with sprains and strains, sea sickness, head injury and abrasions [10]. Fractures and deaths have also been found to occur in people undertaking white-water rafting in New Zealand with 33 fatalities over a 13-year period [22].

*Environmental Locations and Hazards*

While all of these activities occur on water, there are both a range of aquatic locations where the activities are carried out as well as great variability between each type of geographical location. As such, for people to better understand the risk, the American Whitewater Association has classified white water into six difficulty classes [23, 24].

This is not to say all deaths occur in white-water environments and there are a range of hazards faced other than the flow of the water, including interaction with other people and vessels on the water, such as the collision between a kayak and motorboat off the British Virgin Islands in 2002 where an American tourist was killed [25].

Additional hazards faced by paddlers include: environmental hazards such as the temperature of the water, the speed of the water, hitting a submerged objects within the water, colliding with objects such as branches which overhang the water, waterborne diseases, animals (e.g. sharks [26]), the effects of repeated immersion (softening of the skin, blistering, paronychial infections, sinusitis, otitis) and submersion [6, 24, 27–29]; the vessel and associated equipment such as blistering from use of the paddle, cuts and abrasions from contact with the vessel, being hit by another person or their paddle while traversing rapids [6, 24], and from the activity such as overuse injuries, muscle sprains and mechanical injuries (hematomas, lacerations, contusions, concussion, spinal cord injuries and fractures), as well as sustaining slips, trips and fall entering and exiting the vessel and the highest risk of all from drowning due to submersion [6, 24].

## What Is the Outcome?

While rates of deaths due to paddling have been found, they tend to be low. For instance, in 2010 there were 141 fatalities attributable to canoes or kayaks in the USA of which 128 (91%) were due to drowning [15]. Injuries sustained are usually by from striking an object or another person, traumatic stress from the interaction of water, position of the paddler and equipment, overuse injuries and sprains and strains. More often than not these injuries are minor or transient. However, people have been found to dislocate shoulders, fracture parts of the body, and become hypothermic.

Some of the diseases which have also been identified as being acquired while kayaking or rafting include leptospirosis, norovirus and staphylococcal skin infections. Leptospirosis is a bacterial disease caused by a number of different species of the genus *Leptospira*, which causes fever, headaches, muscle pain, nausea, vomiting and bloodshot eyes. If left untreated, people can develop complications and in rare instances these complications can be fatal [30–33]. Leptospirosis has been reported in major studies of returning travellers, such as that from the GeoSentinel Network, but it is not common [34]. There has been a positive link to leptospirosis and participants in adventure sports and exotic tourism in an earlier outbreak reported by the CDC (2001) [35].

The norovirus is a group of viruses that can cause diarrhea, stomach pain and vomiting, although some people may also experience low-grade fever, chills, headache, muscle aches and tiredness. Generally, the symptoms only last 1–2 days. Other names by which the norovirus is known include 'viral gastroenteritis', 'Norwalk-like viruses' and 'stomach flu'. The virus is found in the vomit or feces of infected people and is highly contagious. For instance, people can become infected by ingesting food and drinking liquids which are contaminated, touching a contaminated surface and putting their hand in their mouth, aerosols from projectile vomiting and having contact with another infected person [33, 36, 37].

Decker et al. [38] provided a report on the epidemics of skin infections from *Staphylococcus aureus* while rafting with guides in Tennessee, South Carolina. *S. aureus* or 'golden staph' is a common bacterium that lives in the nose or on the skin. In their study, Decker et al. found that there were two factors contributing to the outbreak – the first factor was frequent minor skin wounds and the second was prolonged close contact to infected individuals. It appears also that cramped living conditions also contributed to the outbreak. Prevention includes washing and showering regularly and use a hexachlorophene scrub solution; people with infections not being allowed to work, nor share quarters and need to seek medical attention, and also the sharing of towels, line and clothing be discouraged.

## What Are the Risk Factors?

A risk factor is those elements associated with an increase in injury or death. As previously describe there is already a classification of the difficulty of the white water (table 3). This provides a measure of the risk for those rivers which have a classification. In order to provide a river with a category a number of the risk factors are used, these include: speed at which the water flows, number and size of hazards (such as rock, trees, etc.), size of the waves, strength of the eddies, water volume, predictability of the rapids, length, and drops or falls in the water level, experience [23, 24].

Other risk factors include: skill level such as the ability to be able to right the vessel (Eskimo roll); experience and familiarity with a particular location; type and familiarity with the equipment being used; need to carry or lift vessel and the weight of the vehicle; water quality; wave height; water temperature; activity being undertaken; sharks or other aquatic animals; wearing of safety equipment; use of alcohol and other drugs, and overloading the vessel [9, 10, 15, 18, 19, 22–24, 26, 28, 30–32].

**Table 3.** Classification of white-water difficulty by the American Whitewater Association, 2011 [24]

| Class | Description |
|---|---|
| Class I: Rapids | Fast-moving water with riffles and small waves. Few obstructions, all obvious and easily missed with little training. Risk to swimmers is slight; self-rescue is easy. |
| Class II: Rapids: novice | Straightforward rapids with wide, clear channels which are evident without scouting. Occasional maneuvering may be required, but rocks and medium-sized waves are easily missed by trained paddlers. Swimmers are seldom injured and group assistance, while helpful, is seldom needed. Rapids that are at the upper end of this difficulty range are designated 'Class II+'. |
| Class III: Intermediate | Rapids with moderate, irregular waves which may be difficult to avoid and which can swamp an open canoe. Complex maneuvers in fast current and good boat control in tight passages or around ledges are often required; large waves or strainers may be present but are easily avoided. Strong eddies and powerful current effects can be found, particularly on large-volume rivers. Scouting is advisable for inexperienced parties. Injuries while swimming are rare; self-rescue is usually easy but group assistance may be required to avoid long swims. Rapids that are at the lower or upper end of this difficulty range are designated 'Class III–' or 'Class III+' respectively. |
| Class IV: Advanced | Intense, powerful but predictable rapids requiring precise boat handling in turbulent water. Depending on the character of the river, it may feature large, unavoidable waves and holes or constricted passages demanding fast maneuvers under pressure. A fast, reliable eddy turn may be needed to initiate maneuvers, scout rapids, or rest. Rapids may require 'must' moves above dangerous hazards. Scouting may be necessary the first time down. Risk of injury to swimmers is moderate to high, and water conditions may make self-rescue difficult. Group assistance for rescue is often essential but requires practiced skills. A strong Eskimo roll is highly recommended. Rapids that are at the lower or upper end of this difficulty range are designated 'Class IV–' or 'Class IV+' respectively. |
| Class 5: Expert | Extremely long, obstructed, or very violent rapids which expose a paddler to added risk. Drops may contain large, unavoidable waves and holes or steep, congested chutes with complex, demanding routes. Rapids may continue for long distances between pools, demanding a high level of fitness. What eddies exist may be small, turbulent, or difficult to reach. At the high end of the scale, several of these factors may be combined. Scouting is recommended but may be difficult. Swims are dangerous, and rescue is often difficult even for experts. A very reliable Eskimo roll, proper equipment, extensive experience, and practiced rescue skills are essential. Because of the large range of difficulty that exists beyond Class IV, Class 5 is an open-ended, multiple-level scale designated by Class 5.0, 5.1, 5.2, etc. – each of these levels is an order of magnitude more difficult than the last. Example: increasing difficulty from Class 5.0 to Class 5.1 is a similar order of magnitude as increasing from Class IV to Class 5.0. |
| Class VI: Extreme and exploratory rapids | These runs have almost never been attempted and often exemplify the extremes of difficulty, unpredictability and danger. The consequences of errors are very severe and rescue may be impossible. For teams of experts only, at favorable water levels, after close personal inspection and taking all precautions. After a Class VI rapids has been run many times, its rating may be changed to an appropriate Class 5.x rating. |

## Injury Prevention

There is very little evidence for the effectiveness of strategies to reduce injuries and deaths from activities associated with paddling, however there is some general advice which is seen as helping to ensure that a person will return safely from paddling trip, this information is provided below. It is recommended that an overall risk management approach be used when any aquatic activity is to be undertaken [39].

The first and foremost protection when undertaking a paddling activity is for a person to wear a lifejacket, in some states this is a mandatory requirement during whitewater activities. A study of recreational boaters who drowned in the USA found that 9 out of 10 were not wearing a lifejacket [15]. Lifejackets come in a variety of sizes and types depending on the conditions and where the activities are being undertaken. In the USA there are five types of lifejacket with type I being the most effective but also has the greatest bulk. Type I lifejackets are designed for open and rough or remote aquatic location where rescue may be slow in coming, they also turn the unconscious wearer face-up in the water and have a high visibility color.

There may also be some opportunities to modify the vessel to improve its resistance to capsizing or where the person is thrown from the vessel or choosing a vessel that is more suited to the skill level of the participant. In a New Zealand study of what causes water rafting deaths, a third (36.4%) were due to the raft overturning/capsizing and another 30.3% were due to the person being thrown out of the raft [22].

Prevention should start before the person even heads out the door, a summary of what should be undertaken prior to commencing a canoeing or kayaking trip can be found in table 4. Ensure that the equipment is in good working order, the lifejacket is not torn, worn, faded (so the person can be seen if they do end up in the water) and is still buoyant and fits properly. Check that the helmet fits and is not worn or cracked. To work properly a lifejacket should fit snugly and not move about the person, particularly for children where it should not allow for the child's chin or ears to slip through.

A plan for the trip should be developed which includes information on where the group are going and when they will be back, where the trip is starting and finishing, where the vehicles will be located, the kayak and lifejacket colors for all the participants, as well as any other information which can help to locate the party faster. The plan should also include contact phone numbers for all participants, emergency services, and the emergency person contact for each participant (e.g. spouse or parent). Ensure that the details of the trip are known by a person not participating so they can send a search party if they do not return. The plan should also include an emergency evacuation procedure and information about what happens if the river conditions change (i.e. there is a downpour which makes the conditions unsafe).

Undertaking a first aid course is also of value not just for this activity but for life in general. Having good resuscitation skills can save a life but there are a lot of injuries sustained where basic first aid cannot only help save a person's life but can also reduce the risk of long-term harm from the injury. A well-equipped first aid kit is also

**Table 4.** Pre-event preparation

| Area | Activity | What to do |
|---|---|---|
| Check equipment | Canoe/kayak | Check it is in working order, no holes, cracks or damage to the craft. |
| | Lifejacket | Ensure it is in working order, still fits, there is no damage, not faded. |
| | Helmet | Check for damage, ensure it is in working order. |
| | Other safety equipment such as distress beacon | Check to ensure they still work, that the batteries are charged and that you have spares. |
| Develop a trip plan | Location | Where will you be going, how are you getting there and where are you parking the vehicles. Where does the trip originate and what is the intended route. |
| | Returning | When will you be coming back. |
| | Who are you going with? | Number of people, names, contact details, vehicle types and registration, canoe/kayak type and color, lifejacket color. |
| | Contact details | Contact details for all the people and who to contact in an emergency is also important. Who has a phone with them and what are the numbers. |
| First aid | Undertake training/ update skills | First aid is a skill for life and everyone should undertake first aid training. Like any skill it needs to be practiced on a regular basis undertake a refresher course at least once a year. |
| | First aid kit | Make sure that you all the essential items, they are not out of date and are in working order. |
| Check conditions | Weather | Ensure you have appropriate sun protection including sunscreen and sunglasses. |
| | River | Ask a local, ranger or someone who visits the area regularly what the conditions are like. Take a trip which matches your skills by checking the white-water difficulty rating. |
| Provisions | Water | Dehydration is a real danger you need to take a gallon of water for each day you are away. |
| | Food | Ensure you have enough for the journey and that it is stored so that it will not become wet if the canoe/kayak capsizes. |
| Training | Technique | Learn proper paddling technique. |
| | Swimming | If you are not a good swimming have a few lesson, go to the local pool and swim a few laps before heading out to check your swimming skills, you will need to swim a few as fitness is an essential part of swimming. |

valuable, and should include bandages, gauze pads, gauze rolls, ibuprofen, iodine, soap, energy bars, rehydration solutions, Dramamine for motion sickness, wrist support in case of tendonitis, sun block, insect repellent, scissors or Swiss army knife with scissors, Steri-Strips, swim ear, Super Glue, waterproof band aids, zip-lock bags, and duct tape. Make sure that the first aid kit is waterproof. Super Glue can also be used for filling blisters – make sure to eliminate as much of the fluid as possible from the blister and glue the loose skin to the skin behind it; the glue does sting on application but after a few minutes it is possible to resume paddling [40].

Immediately before heading out or undertaking the trip, the weather conditions and forecast should be checked for the period of the trip and if necessary plans put in place if rain changes the conditions. Ensure enough drinking water is taken on the trip, the rule of thumb is approximately 1 gallon (4 liters) per day.

Know the river – during the year a river can change depending on the amount of water flowing, be careful when undertaking activities after flooding as the conditions may have changed with boulders and other debris moving due to the large volume of water. Never let people go out alone, if people are rafting for the first time they should be going with an experienced guide, provided with appropriate instruction and ensure the person understands what the guide is saying.

Seek qualified instruction to learn proper paddling techniques prior to commencing and while it is fun to for people to be challenged, ensure that people do not overestimate their own ability. In white-water rafting where predominantly people are using another's service to undertake this activity, ensure that the people providing the activity are responsive to safety, have procedures in place to monitor changes in river conditions, undertake appropriate pre-activity assessment to ensure that participants are matched to the river conditions, know the river and its conditions and have appropriate policies in place for when an activity should be cancelled or discontinued as well as safety or exit points along the journey [39]. If a person is not a good swimmer, they should take some swimming lessons prior to undertaking the activity or go to the pool and swim laps, remember that paddling requires upper body strength and endurance. Know the river classification and choose a classification based on experience, skills, fitness and the physical limitation of the participant.

If a participant does fall out of the canoe, kayak or raft and find themselves being carried along in the water, make sure that they know to float feet first and let the current take them with their feet at the top of the water to stop their feet from getting stuck between rocks, have them move towards the edge of the river when they see a safe exit point. Never try and stand up, the force of the water will push you over.

The prevention of contracting any of the viruses include ensuring that any cuts, grazes and abrasions are dressed in a waterproof dressing, before eating wash hands with disinfectants and ensuring the camping site is clean and tidy to discourage rodents and minimize the contact with animal urine. Clean and disinfect contaminated surfaces immediately.

Other risks include sunburn and hypothermia. Make sure participants are wearing and take with them sunscreen to be reapplied every 2 h, wear clothing that covers as much skin as possible, wear a hat that protects the face, head, neck and ears and also wear sunglasses, they need to remember that they are not only getting exposure directly from the sun but also from the reflection of the water.

Other things to remember are that alcohol and drugs and water do not mix. Alcohol affects coordination, reaction time, judgement and can cause disturbances in the inner ear affecting balance and orientation when in the water, spasm of the vocal cords closing off the airway when in water, and reduces inhibitions and distorts judgement [41]. Statistics from the US Coast Guard show that in 2008 the use of alcohol or drugs, mainly alcohol, was the cause of the greatest number of fatalities [42].

Avoiding collision with other watercraft – ensure that the paddlers are vigilant by watching other boaters and assuming that they cannot see them, this is particularly important where there is a swell where the canoe or kayak may be hidden by the waves. Ensure they follow the rules of the water and avoid shipping channels.

### Further Research

Areas where further research would be of value include: (1) *Definitions* – in this review articles often grouped together paddling activities, or grouped kayaking and canoeing, it would be valuable to define appropriately what is included in these activities, the type of crafts involved, as well as exploring such issues as skill level, equipment and locations. (2) *Epidemiological studies* – while there are a number of studies which have explored injuries and illness to canoeists, kayakers and rafters, there is very little corresponding information on exposure, nor is it clear in many who is the exposed population. (3) *Locations* – the American Whitewater Association has provided a description of the 'international scale of river difficulties' [23, 24], however this information was not used when describing where the deaths or injuries occurred. There was also very little information on actual locations. (4) *Risk factors* – while some of the risk factors have been identified and used in some studies they are not consistently applied or found across all studies and there is a need to better understand the risk factors in order to help develop prevention strategies. (5) *Prevention* – there is a lot of information on the internet about possible prevention activities that could be undertaken.

### Acknowledgements

Richard Franklin is employed by James Cook University as an Associate Professor in Injury Prevention and Safety Promotion, this position is funded by a Queensland Injury Prevention Council academic capacity building grant. He is a Senior Research Fellow with the Royal Life Saving Society, Australia.

## References


1 Simons HJ, Wong CS: The travel health consultation: a focus on risk assessment and risk management. Primary Health Care 2011;21:33–39.

2 Leggat P, Carne J, Kedjarune U: Travel insurance and health. J Travel Med 1999;6:243–248.

3 International Life Saving Federation: Drowning Facts and Figures. URL http://ilsforg/en/drowning/facts (accessed 4 Sept 2011).

4 World Health Organization: Facts about Injuries: Drowning. Geneva, WHO, 2003; URL. http://www.who.int/violence_injury_prevention/publications/other_injury/en/drowning_factsheet.pdf (accessed 4 Sept 2011).

5 Leggat P, Wilks G: Overseas visitor deaths in Australia, 2001–2003. J Travel Med 2009;16:243–247.

6 Shepard R: Science and medicine of canoeing and kayaking. Sports Med 1987;4:19–33.

7 Outdoor Foundation: Outdoor recreation: participation report. A look at trends in American participation in outdoor recreation with a focus on youth, diversity and the future of the outdoors. Outdoor Foundation. 2010; http://www.outdoorfoundation.org/research.participation.2010.html (accessed 4 Sept 2010).

8 Outdoor Industry Association, Outdoor Foundation: A special report on paddle sports, 2009: kayaking, canoeing and rafting. Outdoor Industry Association and Outdoor Foundation. 2009; http://www.outdoorfoundation.org/research.paddlesports.html (accessed 4 Sept 2010).

9 Jackson DM, Verscheure SK: Back pain in whitewater rafting guides. Wilderness Environ Med 2006; 17:162–170.

10 Bailey I: An analysis of sea kayaking incidents in New Zealand 1992–2005. Wilderness Environ Med 2010;21:208–218.

11 US Coast Guard: Department of Homeland Security (US): Recreational Boating Statistics – 2006: US Coast Guard. 2007; URL. http://www.uscgboating.org/assets/1/Publications/Boating_Statistics_2006.pdf (accessed 4 Sept 2011).

12 US Coast Guard: Department of Homeland Security (US): Recreational Boating Statistics – 2007. US Coast Guard. 2008; URL. http://www.uscgboating.org/assets/1/Publications/Boating_Statistics_2007.pdf (accessed 4 Sept 2011).

13 US Coast Guard: Department of Homeland Security (US): Recreational Boating Statistics – 2008. US Coast Guard. 2009; URL. http://www.uscgboating.org/assets/1/Publications/Boating_Statistics_2008.pdf (accessed 4 Sept 2011).

14 US Coast Guard: Department of Homeland Security (US): Recreational Boating Statistics – 2009. US Coast Guard. 2010; URL. http://www.uscgboating.org/assets/1/workflow_staging/Publications/394.pdf (accessed 4 Sept 2011).

15 US Coast Guard: Department of Homeland Security (US): Recreational Boating Statistics – 2010. US Coast Guard. 2011; URL. http://www.uscgboating.org/assets/1/workflow_staging/Page/2010_Recreational_Boating_Statistics.pdf (accessed 4 Sept 2011).

16 Wittmann L: Kayaking is safer than you might think (really!). American Whitewater 2000(Sept-Oct): 100–101.

17 Mason M: West Virginia whitewater stays the course for 30 years. Charleston Gaz 1998(Aug 2):1c, 5c.

18 Whisman SA, Hollenhorst SJ: Injuries in commercial whitewater rafting. Clin J Sport Med 1999;9: 18–23.

19 Kameyama O, Shibana K, Kawakita H, Ogawa R, Kumamoto M: Medical check of competitive canoeists. J Orthop Sci 1999;4:243–249.

20 Powell C: Injuries and Medical conditions among kayakers paddling in the sea environment. Wilderness Environ Med 2009;20:237–334.

21 Krupnick J, Cox R, Summers R: Injuries sustained during competitive white-water paddling: a survey of athletes in the 1996 Olympic trials. Wilderness Environ Med 1998;9:14–18.

22 O'Hare D, Chalmers D, Arnold NA, Williams F: Mortality and morbidity in white water rafting in New Zealand. Inj Control Saf Promot 2002;9:193–198.

23 American Whitewater. IV. International Scale of River Difficulty; in Safety Code of American Whitewater. Adopted 1959, revised 2005. http://wwwamericanwhitewaterorg/content/Wiki/do-op/id/safety%3Astart/#vi_international_scale_of_river_difficulty. 2005 (accessed 4 Sept 2011).

24 Fiore DC: Injuries associated with whitewater rafting and kayaking. Wilderness Environ Med 2003; 14:255–260.

25 Joyst Van Dyke, British Virgin Islands. URL http://jostvandykeco/about/kayaking-and-hiking (accessed 4 Sept 2011).

26 Kizer K: Shark and other aquatic predator attacks on kayakers. Wilderness Environ Med 2011;22:100–101.

27 Fiore DC, Houston J: Injuries in whitewater kayaking. Br J Sports Med 2001;35:235–241.

28 Kizer K: Medical aspects of white-water kayaking. Phys Sports Med 1987;15:128–137.

29 Schoen R, Stano M: Year 2000 whitewater injury survey. Wilderness Environ Med 2002;13:119–124.
30 Blackburn BMD: Leptospirosis in Florida: recreational exposures herald new serovars and highlight environmental impact. Infect Dis Alert 2011;30: 64–66.
31 Centers for Disease Control: Outbreak of leptospirosis among white-water rafters: Costa Rica, 1996. MMWR Morb Mortal Wkly Rep 1997;46: 577–579.
32 Stephan C, Hunfeld KP, Schonberg A, Ott MG, Hetzenecker M, Bitzer R, et al: Leptospirosis after a staff outing (in German, Engl. Abstr.). Dtsch Med Wochenschr 2000;125:623–627.
33 Heymann D (ed): Control of Communicable Diseases Manual, ed 19. Washington, American Public Health Association, 2008.
34 Freedman D, Weld L, Kozarsky P, et al: Spectrum of disease and relation to place of exposure amongst ill returned travellers. N Engl J Med 2006;354:119–130.
35 Centers for Disease Control and Prevention: Update: outbreak of acute febrile illness amongst athletes participating in Eco-Challenge, Sabah 2000, Borneo, Malaysia, 2000. MMWR Morb Mortal Wkly Rep 2001;50:21–24.
36 Jones EL, Gaither M, Kramer A, Gerba CP: An analysis of water quality in the Colorado River, 2003–2004; an investigation into recurring outbreaks of norovirus among rafters. Wilderness Environ Med 2009;20:6–13.
37 Malek M, Barzilay E, Kramer A, Camp B, Jaykus L-A, Escudero-Abarca B, et al: Outbreak of norovirus infection among river rafters associated with packaged delicatessen meat, Grand Canyon, 2005. Clin Infect Dis 2009;48:31–37.
38 Decker M, Lybarger J, Vaughn W, Hutcheson R, Schaffner W: An outbreak of staphylococcal skin infections among river rafting guides. Am J Epidemiol 1986;124:969–976.
39 Hunter IR: An analysis of whitewater rafting safety data: risk management for programme organizers. J Adventure Educ Outdoor Learn 2007;7:21–35.
40 Stone J: What's up doc? The first aid kit. Paddle World. 2011;http://www.paddleworld.com/first-aid-kayak.php (accessed 4 Sept 2011).
41 Chellew C, Franklin RC, Simmonds E: Swim safe, swim sober: a study examining drowning in NSW and the influence of alcohol. Sydney, The Royal Life Saving Society Australia/NSW Branch, 2009.
42 Tomczuk S, Maxim L: Recreational boating accidents statistics and trends. Clear progress, but work remains. US Coast Guard, 2010.

Prof. Peter A. Leggat
School of Public Health, Tropical Medicine and Rehabilitation Sciences
James Cook University
Townsville, QLD 4811 (Australia)
Tel. +61 7 4781 6108, E-Mail peter.leggat@jcu.edu.au

Heggie TW, Caine DJ (eds): Epidemiology of Injury in Adventure and Extreme Sports.
Med Sport Sci. Basel, Karger, 2012, vol 58, pp 112–129

# The Epidemiology of Injury in Bungee Jumping, BASE Jumping, and Skydiving

Kjetil Søreide

Department of Surgery, Stavanger University Hospital, and Institute of Health and Medicine, University of Stavanger, Stavanger, Norway

**Abstract**

Knowledge regarding epidemiology of injury is of benefit to injury prevention of activities associated with high risk. As relatively 'young' activities, the investigation of injuries and deaths related in extreme sports such as bungee jumping and BASE jumping is relatively sparse. Studies evaluating risk in civilian and military skydiving activities have been reported over the past decades, but technique and equipment has changed. Risk with bungee jumping is only sporadically reported in the literature, most often in connection with eye injuries, but also rare events of serious, life-threatening injuries and even death. BASE is an acronym for Building, Antenna, Span, Earth, which represents the fixed objects from which jumps are made. Estimated risk in BASE jumping for any injury (independent of severity grade) is 0.4–0.5%, which as 5- to 8-fold higher than skydiving. Typically, men outnumber women in a ratio of 10:1 in both injuries and case fatality rates. Age is frequently reported to range from 30 to 40 years. Notably, differences in training and environmental locations exist between recreational skydiving and BASE jumping. As BASE jumps are made from lower altitudes than skydives, jumpers generally fall at lower speeds, have far less aerodynamic control, and may lose flying stability. Yet, typical injuries include a bruised or sprained ankle during landing. Protective gear including helmet and pads may help to prevent such injuries, while more complex knowledge of human factors, environment and training are needed to prevent fatal injuries.



Worldwide, risk-associated activity has never been more popular [1]. Together with risk-taking activity, such as airborne sports activities, comes the chance for injuries, disability, and even death [2–9]. Indeed, risk-taking behavior is associated with trauma in general [10, 11]. Thus, knowledge about patterns of injury and death is of benefit in activities associated with high risk. As relatively 'young' activities, the investigation of injuries and deaths related to extreme sports such as bungee jumping and BASE jumping is relatively sparse. In contrast, studies evaluating risk in civilian and military skydiving activities have been reported in the past, but technique and equipment have changed. For example, parachute jumping during the 1970s and 1980s was performed with round canopies packed in bulky harnesses with belly-mounted reserves. These were later replaced by steerable wing parachutes with the main and reserve parachutes both packed into one compact backpack. Thus, skydiving studies from the past cannot immediately be compared to present activity and reports. There is clearly a need for more investigation into these fields of risk taking activity, and this chapter will seek to review the epidemiology of injury related to bungee jumping, BASE jumping, and skydiving, and to provide suggestions for further research.

## Methods

This chapter is based on a search of the literature in PubMed/Medline over the last decade (2000–2011) with a strong emphasis on reports from the last 5 years (until August 2011). Older references are included where evidence or reports are otherwise scarce. The reference lists of articles identified by this search strategy were also searched and articles judged relevant were also selected. Studies are primarily related to civilian activity, as reports from military parachute activity may not allow for immediate comparison [12–17]. Searches were performed using the index words 'BASE jumping' or 'Bungee jumping' or 'Skydiving' with 'injury', 'risk' or 'mortality'. Secondary internet resources, including Google Scholar, Wikipedia and related homepages were searched for information where appropriate for the topic.

## Brief Historic Overview and Definitions

The history of risk-taking activity and extreme sports dates back several centuries. Concerning the topics related to this chapter, the activity called 'bungee' (or 'bungy') jumping is probably the oldest. In the 1950s, David Attenborough and a BBC film crew brought back footage of the 'land divers' (known as *Naghol*) of the Pentecost Island in Vanuatu/South Pacific, young men who jumped from tall wooden platforms with vines tied to their ankles as a test of their courage and passage into manhood. A similar practice, only with a much slower pace for falling, has been practiced as the *Danza de los Voladores de Papantla* or the 'Papantla flyers' of Central Mexico, a tradition dating back to the days of the Aztecs. The first 'modern' bungee jumps were made on April 1, 1979, from a 76-meter suspension bridge in Bristol by the Oxford University Dangerous Sports Club [18]. Commercial bungee jumping began with the New Zealander, Alan J. Hackett, who made his first jump from Auckland's Greenhithe Bridge in 1986. The first injuries related to this sport was reported only two decades ago [19].

BASE is an acronym for Building, Antenna, Span, Earth, and thus represents the fixed objects from which BASE jumps are made [6–9]. BASE jumping is in general regarded as an 'extreme sport', with a calculated risk of serious injury or even death

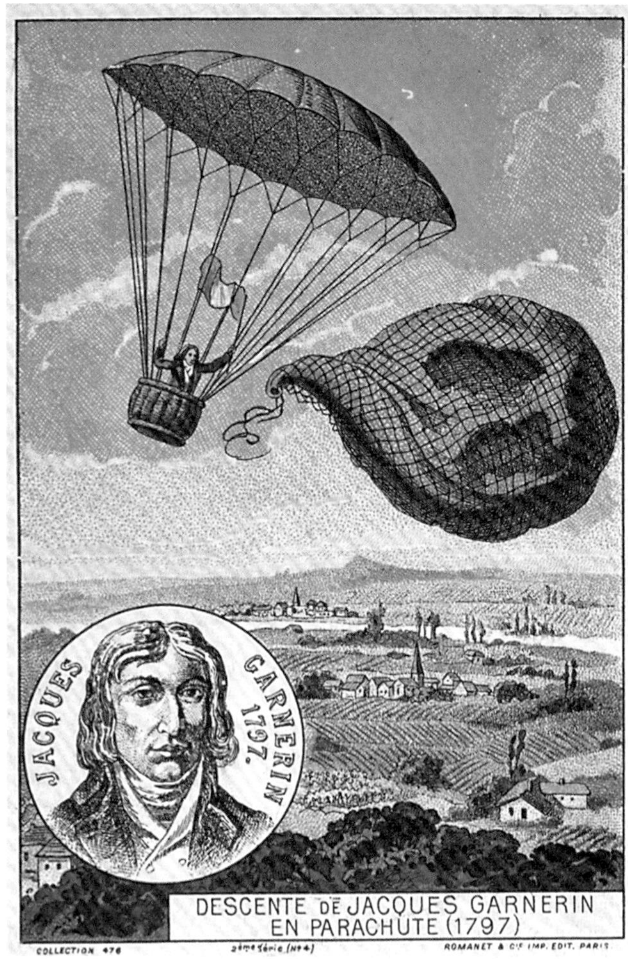


**Fig. 1.** First parachute jump: Garnerin releases the balloon and descends with the help of a parachute, 1797. Illustration from the late 19th century [from Wikipedia, no copyrights attached].

involved. Consequently, and to ensure public safety, BASE jumping has been banned from most public places, including popular attractions such as the Eiffel Tower in Paris, France. Furthermore, BASE jumping has spurred critique as it may be potentially hazardous not only for those involved, but, also for the emergency medicine service (EMS) involved in rescue, as it may be performed in remote areas with difficult access for rescue workers [8]. Nonetheless, BASE jumping has grown in magnitude and activity and it is estimated that more than 35,000 jumps are performed annually in Norway alone (unpublished report). Further, new developments in equipment, such as wingsuits have given rise to new terms and activities, such as WiSBASE (wingsuit BASE jumping) of which few or no injury or mortality statistics are found particularly.

The history of skydiving starts with Andre-Jacques Garnerin (fig. 1) who made successful parachute jumps from a hot-air balloon. He carried out the first jump with a silk parachute in 1797 at Parc Monceau, in Paris/France. The military developed parachuting technology as a way to save aircrews from emergencies aboard balloons and aircraft in flight, later as a way of delivering soldiers to the battlefield. Early competitions date back to the 1930s, and it became an international sport in 1952.

### Who Is Affected by Injury?

Although millions of jumps have been performed over the latter half century, there is only limited reporting and data on injuries, risks and fatalities in these activities. For bungee jumping, research is limited to case reports and a few case series, and an absence of cross-sectional or cohort research.

For BASE jumping there are but a few studies, although some new data has emerged over the last several years [6–9, 20]. An estimated risk in BASE jumping for any injury (independent of severity grade) is based on two studies, one from Norway and the other from New Zealand, both arriving at an estimate of 0.4–0.5%, or 1 injury in every 200 jumps [7, 8]. The risk associated with BASE jumping is 5- to 8-fold higher than that reported for regular skydiving [7–9, 21].

Skydiving is somewhat more thoroughly investigated [2–4, 21–23]. Risk in skydiving has been estimated to about 5 deaths and 140–170 injuries per 100,000 parachute jumps [3, 5]. However, substantial changes and evolvement in training, equipment and experience over past decades prevents meaningful comparison with more recent research relative to risk, injury or mortality statistics (fig. 2).

### Where Does Injury Occur?

*Anatomical Location*

For bungee jumping the data are based on case reports or small case series. The most frequent injury is to the eyes such as retinal bleeding from the increased intravascular pressure during the bungee recoil [24–35]. Acute venous stasis in the head may include skin edema, purpura-like bleeding in the face and the conjunctiva, dizziness, confusion and transient visual problems [36]. However, other injuries have been described ranging from extremity fractures and dislocations [37, 38] to carotid vascular injury with the consequence of stroke (cerebral insult) [39], severe neck injury with quadriplegia and lastly, fatal outcomes [40]. Further, bungee jumping has been shown to increase stress and decrease immune function at the molecular level [41, 42].

Spinal injuries, for the most being compression fractures, are reported in 30–50% of incidents in BASE jumping and skydiving [6, 20]. This is 3–5 times more frequent than spinal injuries seen in populations of general trauma [43], and reflects an increase risk for this injury pattern with these airborne activities.

Patterns of injury reported in Swedish skydivers [21] are depicted in figure 3 and involve primarily the extremities, back/spine and head, with most injuries being low-

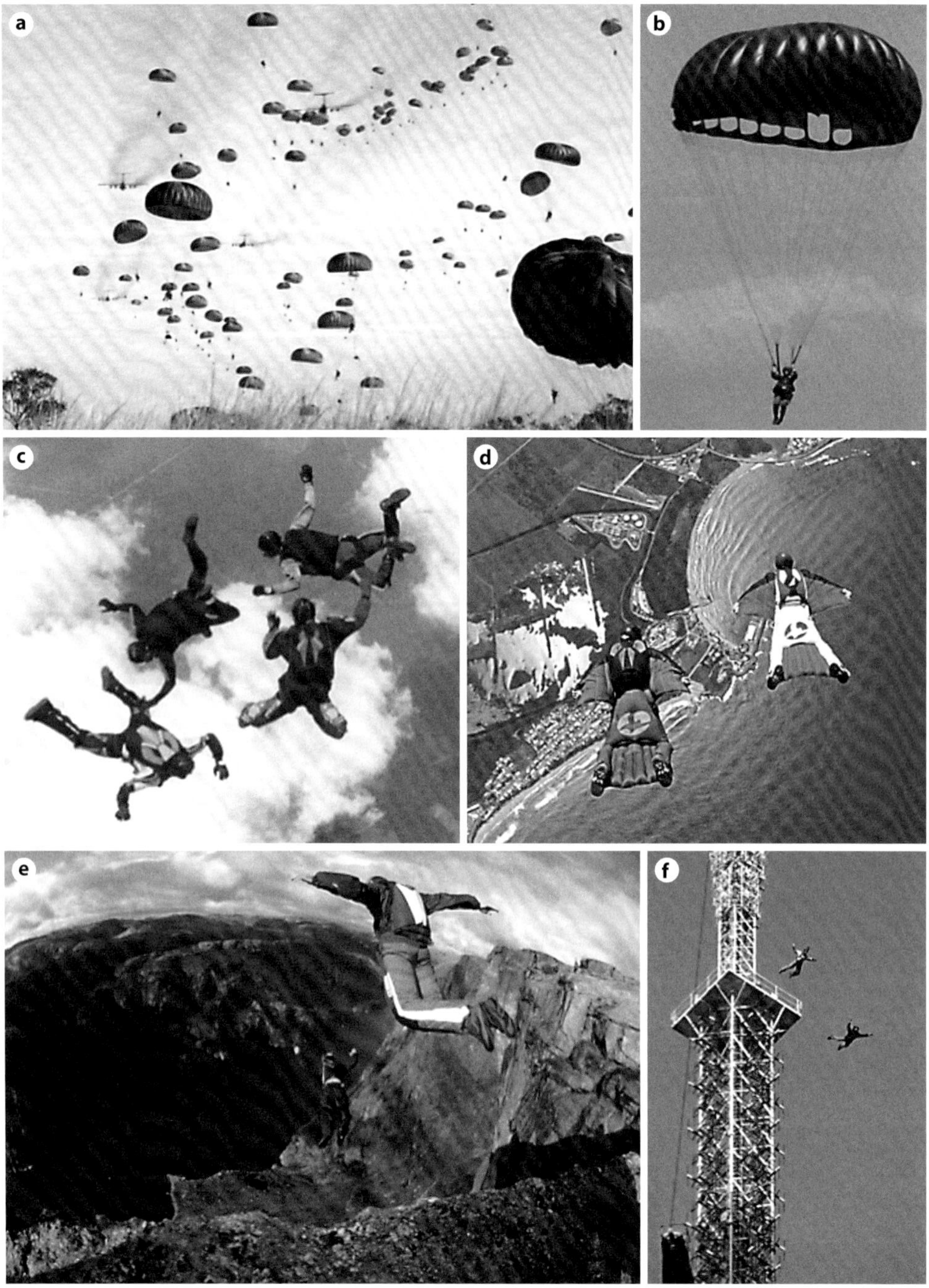

**Fig. 2.** Different types of parachute activity and techniques.

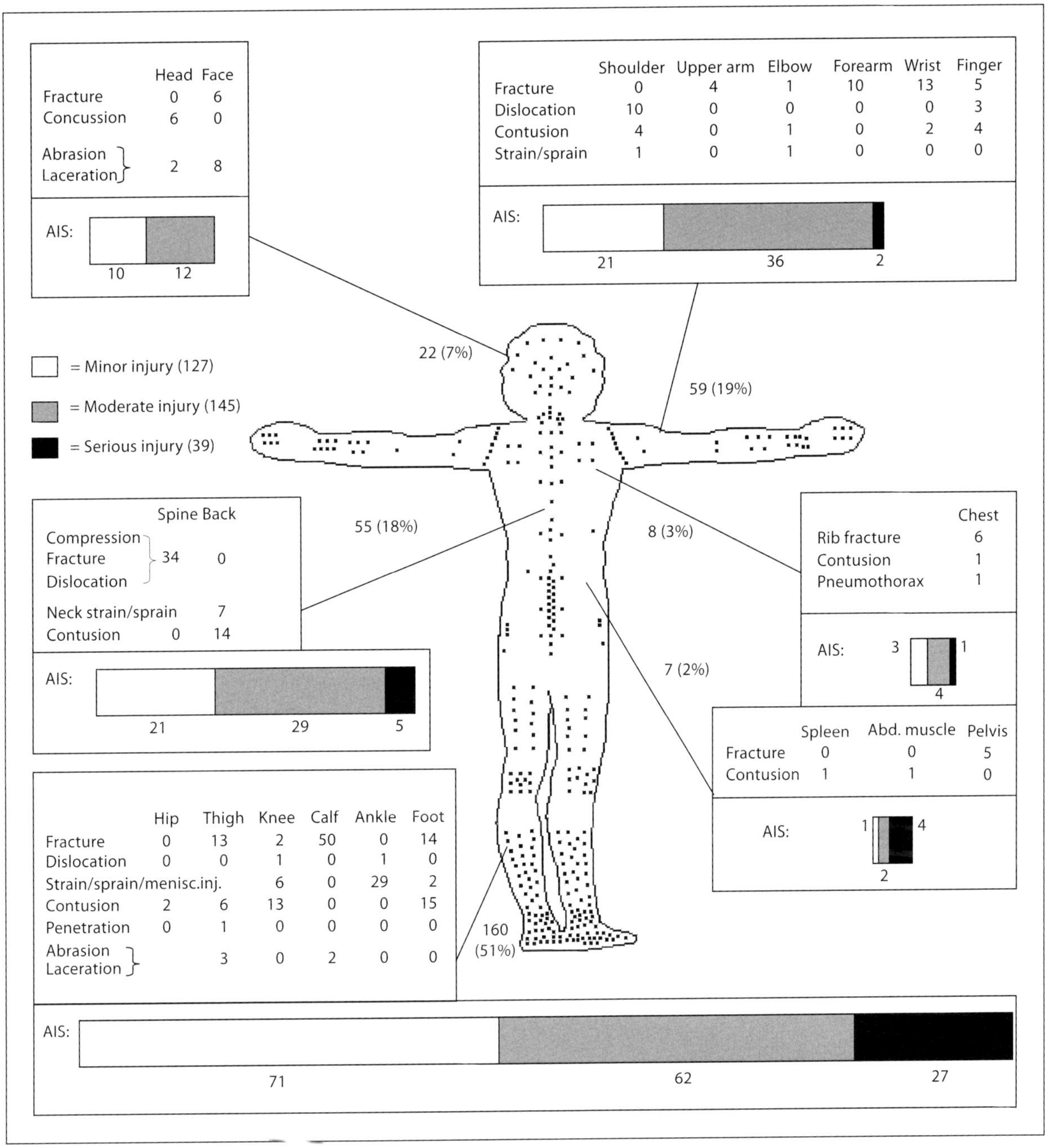


**Fig. 3.** Patterns of injury reported in Swedish skydivers [reproduced from Westman et al., Br J Sports Med, 2007, with permission].

grade or minor. Similar patterns are described in other skydiving activities including BASE jumps [6, 7], but immediate comparison is not possible, and data are too scarce to draw firm conclusions.

*Environmental Location*

Adverse events occur more frequently in untrained or inexperienced jumpers, and when not paying heed to local weather conditions [13, 16, 17, 44, 45]. Although not reported in detail here, the impression is that minor or moderate adverse events that occur with BASE jumping are similar in magnitude, cause, and consequence as those associated with civilian or military parachute jumping [46–49]. Typically, they involve a sprained or fractured ankle, minor head concussion, or a bruised/strained knee in association with landing [13, 17, 23, 45, 46].

Notably, some differences in the environmental locations are inherited in the nature of the activity and as such differ between regular skydiving and BASE jumping (fig. 4). As BASE jumps are made from lower altitudes than skydives (often less than 500 ft above ground level), BASE jumpers generally fall at lower speeds, have far less aerodynamic control, and may lose flying stability. Further, if the parachute is deployed while the jumper is unstable there is a high risk of entanglement or malfunction. The single canopy used may also be facing the wrong direction. Such an off-heading opening is not problematic in skydiving, but off-heading opening that results in object strike is the leading cause of serious injury and death in BASE jumping. Also as BASE jumping takes place in close proximity to a cliff or tower which provides the jump platform, the BASE jumper may collide with the object.

The Kjerag Massif in Norway (fig. 2e), although highly challenging, may not pose near as high a risk as BASE jumps from other sites. In particular, this will be true for places where jumping is illegal (i.e. public buildings, skyscrapers, city antennae), for jumps performed during dusk or dawn when lighting may be suboptimal, or even jumps performed when under the influence of drugs or alcohol. Bad judgment may dramatically increase the hazards in risk-taking activity, and thus there is potential for an adverse outcome. However, registration of illegal activity is unlikely, and thus open, well-organized, legally permitted BASE sites such as Kjerag will have to benchmark the risk associated with BASE jumping.

In contrast, one study from the USA reported an increase in landing-related fatalities in modern skydiving, most likely attributed to newer and better equipment that allowed for more aggressive flying [23].

## When Does Injury Occur?

*Injury Onset*

It is likely that the vast majority of injuries in bungee jumping, BASE jumping, and skydiving, are sudden onset or acute injuries. However, few data are available which

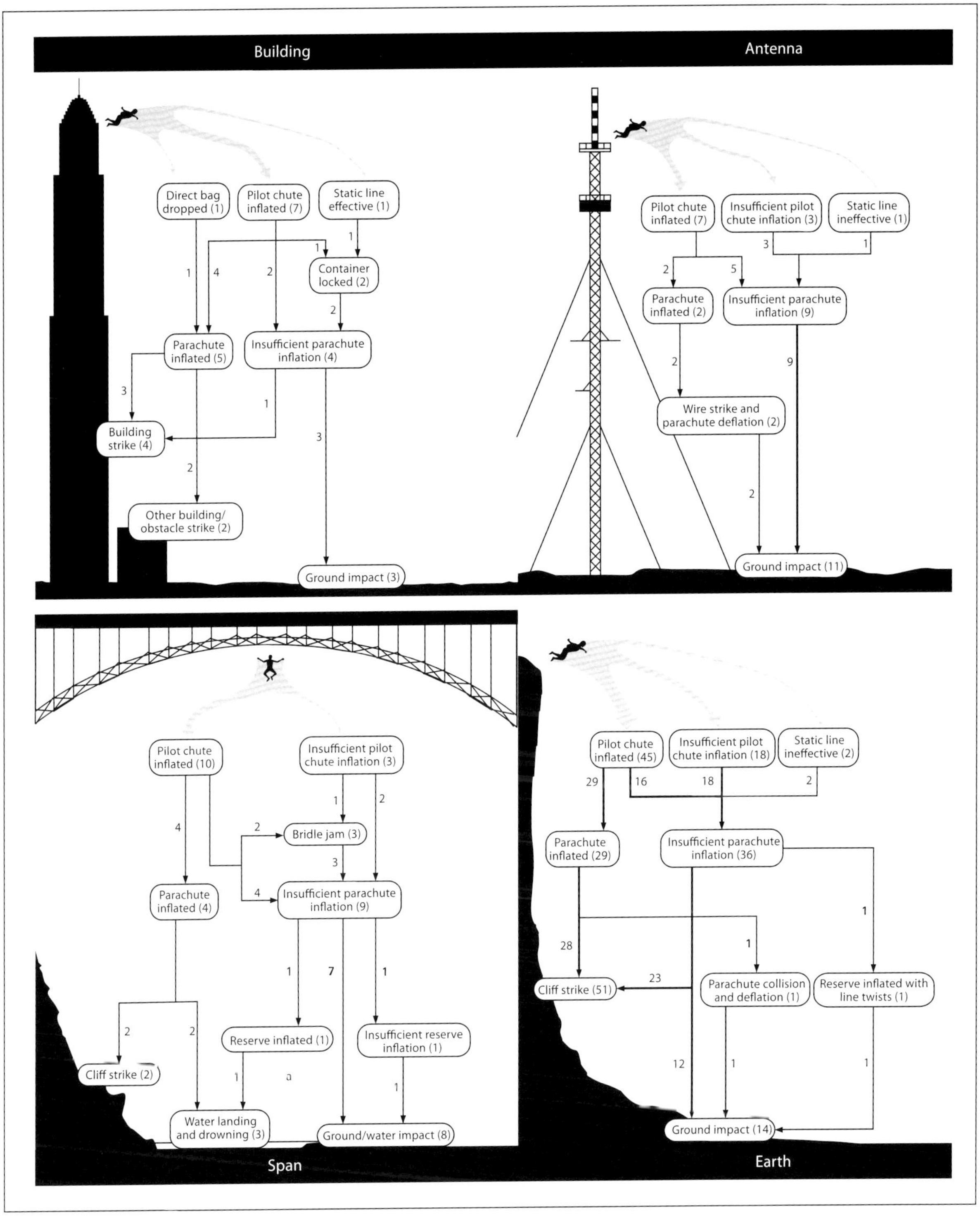


**Fig. 4.** Case fatality analysis in BASE jumping [reproduced from Westman et al., Br J Sports Med, 2008, with permission].

relate to onset of injury in these sports. Knowingly, for bungee jumpers this may often be a one-time experience.

*Chronometry*

There are few data on the 'timing' of injuries in bungee jumping, BASE jumping, and skydiving. Not surprisingly, there is an increased frequency of all injuries during the period of year with most activity, i.e. from April/May until August/September [8, 21]. Although the incidence of fatal injuries in regular skydiving has dropped since the 1960 to the 2000s [2], there appears to be an association between number of jumps and adverse events in both skydiving (fig. 5) and BASE jumping (fig. 6), at least as reported in the past [8].

## What Is the Outcome?

*Injury Type*

For bungee jumping the injury types are limited to case reports, of which ocular manifestations of temporal visual loss due to retinal hemorrhage appears as one of the most frequently reported medical problems [25–29, 31–35, 50]. Also, musculoskeletal and neurological injuries have been described [38, 51], as well as damage to vessels of the neck and intracerebral bleeding [39, 52, 53]. Altogether, reports are scarce and likely underreporting causes a bias in interpretation of these events.

The injury types associated with BASE jumping and skydiving are fairly similar by nature and involve the musculoskeletal system, typically involving minor bruises of ankles, knees and/or a head concussion [7–9, 21]. Fractures in lower and upper extremities may occur (again, typically, ankles, legs, arms/wrists), and injury types and severity may be severe across several body regions when fatal outcomes are reported [2, 4, 8, 20].

*Injury Severity*

In bungee jumping, most visual symptoms reported are self-limiting although blindness and loss of visual acuity has been reported [26, 27, 32–35]. The majority of injuries sustained in skydiving and BASE jumping are characterized as mild to moderate (in about 66% of cases) and sustained in the musculoskeletal system as ankle, knee and shoulder injuries [3], either requiring no or only ambulant medical care, or in some cases in-hospital care (i.e. for fracture treatment, or the like). Fatalities occur in about 0.04% of all BASE jumps, and at much lower rates for recreational skydiving activities [3, 21, 54].

*Clinical Outcome*

No specific data on outcome after minor or moderate injuries exist for these. However, on a general note, the outcome and function after, for example, a fractured ankle may

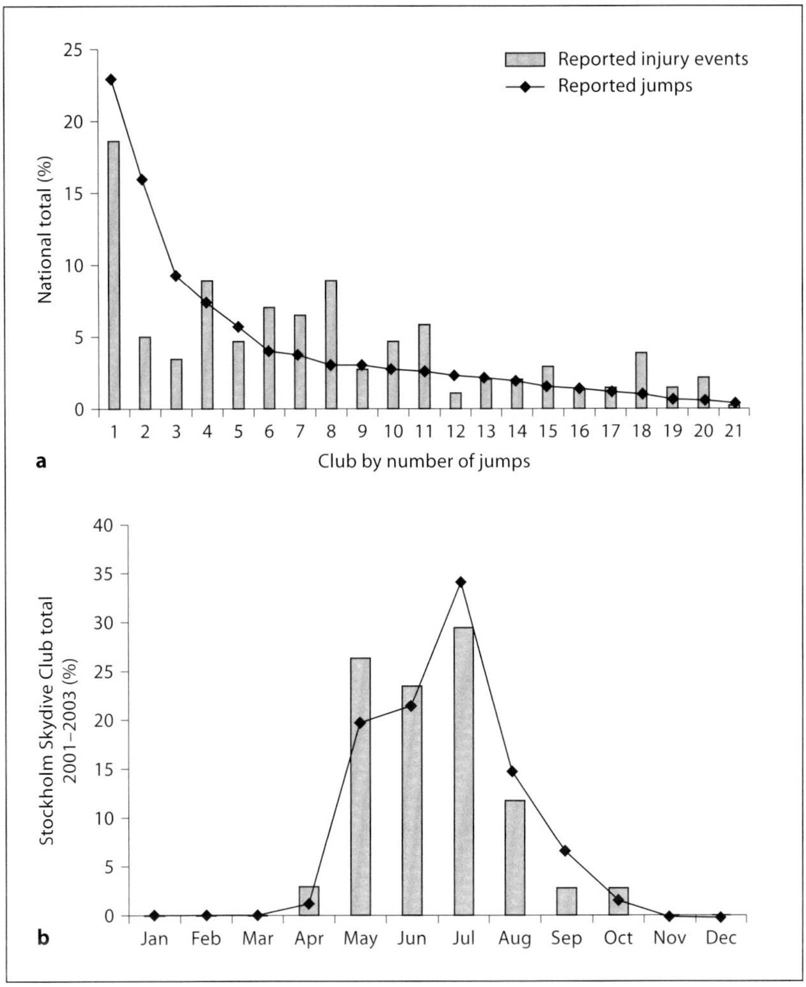


**Fig. 5.** Incidence and seasonal onset of injuries in skydiving. **a** The number of jumps and events for different clubs as reported in Sweden. **b** The temporal association with a monthly predisposition to 'summertime' for most incidents [reproduced from Westman et al., from Br J Sports Med, with permission].

represent the same time off work and in recovery as similar injuries sustained by other mechanisms. It is thus not possible to specifically account outcomes after these injuries other than those reported for all such injuries in a general trauma population.

Cases of quadriplegia or death are noted in bungee jumping, although rare [19]. Intracerebral hemorrhage has been noted on a few occasions, although also infrequently [39, 52, 53].

Fatal outcome has been reported in BASE jumping, and a web-page report on consecutive fatalities known to the BASE jumper enthusiast globally, but may not be complete [55]. At the time of writing it includes descriptions of 164 case fatalities, many

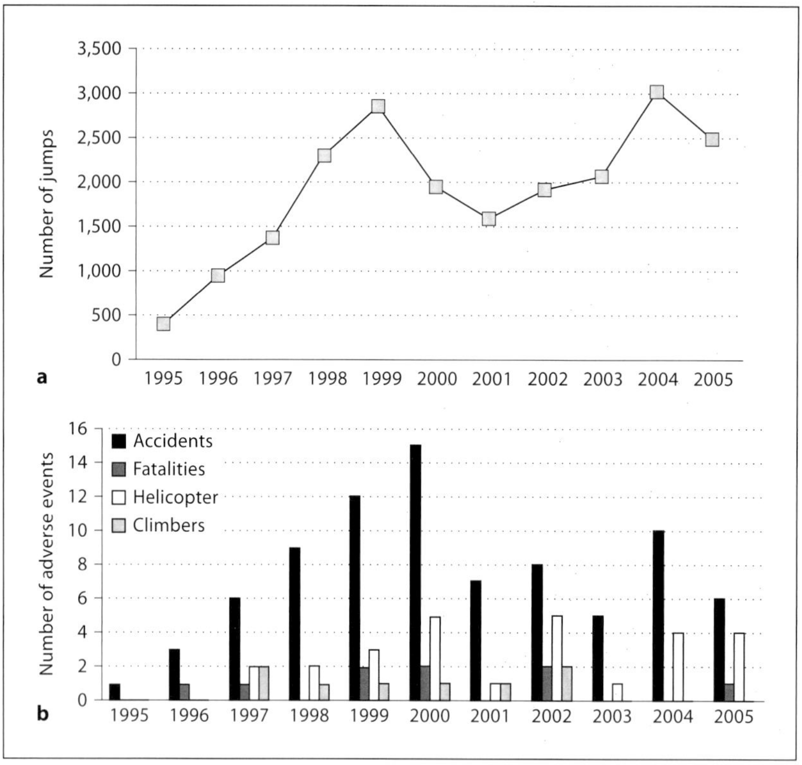


**Fig. 6.** Correlation of (**a**) jumping frequency and (**b**) adverse events in BASE jumping [reproduced with permission from Soreide et al., J Trauma, 2007 with permission].

of which occurred in the USA, Switzerland, Norway, Italy and France [55]. Although this list may not be complete, or contain exact data for each event, it does represent a learning opportunity for the BASE community and highlights possible pitfalls and areas for prevention specific to the cites described.

In the USA alone, an estimated 30–40 deaths occur annually due to skydiving [4]. Fatal injuries are most often sustained to multiple body regions, including head, thorax and abdomen, as well as to extremities. Forensic description of such injuries is scarce, and limited to one case report related to BASE jumping [20]. However, an analysis of 10 BASE-jumping deaths reported in 2007, noted combinations of several severe injuries in multiple body regions; many of the isolated injuries could have been fatal alone [8]. This finding reflects the mechanism and energy transfer associated with such injuries, often caused by object or ground impact in failed jumping attempts.

*Economic Cost*

Information related to cost of treatment associated with injuries, and school or working time loss as a result of injury is virtually non-existent in regard to bungee jumping and BASE. However, past studies have reported considerable health costs associated with injuries sustained from parachute jumping [47, 56]. One critical UK study even stated that parachute jumping for charity purposes actually cost the NHS (National Health Service) 13 times as much as each charitable pound received [56].

For BASE jumping, the local EMS may need activation in the case of an adverse event or injury occurring in remote areas. As reported for the Kjerag Massif in Norway [8], the local EMS is influenced by adverse events associated with BASE jumping. The helicopter EMS responded in one third of all adverse events, and clearly helicopter EMS activity increased with number of accidents, which again followed the annual increase in jumps (fig. 6). Although this study could not specifically address injuries requiring admission to the hospital outpatient or emergency departments, or costs associated with hospital stay or treatment, the activation of the EMS is costly per se. Future investigation should include data that permit description of injury spectrum and severity, treatment requirements, and cost-related estimates for each incident involved with BASE jumps.

## What Are the Risk Factors?

Westman et al. [9] reviewed 100 case fatalities from the 'BASE fatality list' and reported the summarized findings. Human factors included parachutist free-fall instability (loss of body control before parachute deployment), free-fall acrobatics and deployment failure by the parachutist (fig. 4). Equipment factors included pilot chute malfunction and parachute malfunction. In cliff jumping (BASE object type E), parachute opening towards the object jumped was the most frequent equipment factor. Environmental factors included poor visibility, strong or turbulent winds, cold and water. The overall annual fatality risk for all object types during the year 2002 was estimated at about 1 fatality per 60 participants [9].

### *Intrinsic Factors*

Typically, men outnumber women in a ratio of almost 10:1 in both skydiving and BASE-jumping injuries and case fatalities [2, 8, 9, 21]. Age is frequently reported to range from 30 to 40 years in all three sports, which reflects the relatively young yet mature population of people involved in these activities.

### *Extrinsic Factors*

In North American reports [4, 23, 54], landing errors were responsible for most of the skydiving fatalities in more experienced skydivers. The United States Parachute Association (USPA) states that this is due to a new generation of parachutes with higher wing loading [57]. Using data on fatalities from 1992 to 2005 as reported by the USPA [57], hook turns were found to be a major cause of death but not significantly associated with higher wing loading. Fatalities caused by not having a functional parachute have decreased over the years, possibly due to introduction and widespread use of safety devices.

Table 1. Taxonomy by Hart and Griffin [23]

| Categories of fatality | |
|---|---|
| **Fatality category** | **Category definition** |
| No pull/ low pull | Fatalities caused by the failure to pull parachute deployment handles or by deployment that was initiated at an altitude too low for successful inflation of the parachute |
| Landing | Fatalities caused by a conscious skydiver colliding with the ground or an object on the ground while under a fully deployed, undamaged parachute |
| Gear failure | Fatalities resulting from a mechanical or structural failure of gear |
| Incorrect gear | Fatalities caused by the incorrect donning or configuring of gear |
| Midair collision | Fatalities caused by a midair collision during free-fall or under parachutes |
| Medical | Fatalities directly caused by some medical condition such as a heart attack. Also included in this category are clear-cut cases of suicide, e.g., suicide note |
| Incorrect procedures | Fatalities caused by pulling parachute deployment or disconnect handles in an incorrect sequence during normal deployment or following a main parachute malfunction |
| Correct procedures | Fatalities which occurred as the result of failed parachute deployments, despite correct procedures |
| Collapse | Fatalities resulting from a parachute collapse at an altitude too low for corrective action |
| Flight | Fatalities resulting from parachute control inputs that result in canopy failure or loss of control at an altitude too low for corrective action |

A combination of intrinsic and extrinsic factors may be involved in all aspects of skydiving events. Whether exiting the aircraft, falling with other jumpers, deploying the parachute, dealing with malfunctions, or landing, there are opportunities for errors and failures that are potentially fatal. Fatalities have involved falling out of a parachute harness that was not securely fastened, diving into the spinning propeller of a trailing aircraft, and failing to pull the appropriate release handles when the main parachute did not open properly [54, 57].

A proposed taxonomy for classifying fatal events after skydiving has been proposed and revised by Hart and Griffith [4, 23, 54] (table 1). This has been used by other investigators but with small numbers [2]. Nonetheless, it gives a reasonable standard against which investigators can judge and investigate the events into categories involving human errors or errors due to equipment or technique, and which may find areas for improvement and for future prevention of similar events. A similar analysis was done for BASE-jumping fatalities by Westman et al. [9].

## What Are the Inciting Events?

Bungee-jumping injuries may be divided into those that occur secondary to equipment mishap or tragic accidents, and those that occur regardless of safety measures. In the first instance, injury can happen if the safety harness fails, the cord elasticity is miscalculated, or the cord is not properly connected to the jump platform [58, 59]. Ocular injuries that occur despite safety measures generally relate to the abrupt rise in upper body intravascular pressure during bungee cord recoil.

Similarly, inciting events related to BASE jumping and skydiving may be related to equipment (failure of equipment; wrong equipment; failed use of equipment) or factors related to human error (poor judgment related to location, weather, equipment use, etc.).

## Injury Prevention

Few injury prevention measures have been tested in the sports of bungee jumping, BASE jumping, and skydiving. Proper preparation and training is mandatory for all aspects of risk-taking activity. Some safety measures may indeed prevent or reduce injury or advertent outcomes in the case of an accident takes place.

*Bungee Jumping*

In a case of bungee jumping where the elastic cord broke, or the harness failed, a major casualty was prevented from a 240 ft free fall by having an air cushion on the ground below [59]. This may not always be practically available, and the type of ground surface and height of free fall may thus be determining in the type and outcome of injury.

*BASE Jumping*

Fundamental in preventing injuries is training, experience, and adherence to advice from local and experienced BASE jumpers. Deaths in the Kjerag study [8] occurred in jumpers from different nations with varying degrees of experience in skydiving and BASE jumping (data not reported). All deaths had multiple, severe injuries to several body regions. However, even otherwise survivable injuries (i.e. hemorrhage from fractures) may be fatal when sustained in this extremely challenging environment – a fact that those involved in risk-taking should not ignore. As opposed to other reports [2], no deaths were caused by drowning. To keep the risk of drowning to a minimum, a lifeboat is present during all jumping activity. In order to further reduce adverse events, instruction and training within the BASE community is imperative. A mandatory instructional course is now held for all BASE jumpers at the Kjerag Massif. Continuously, preventive work and safety precautions are implemented in order to reduce the risk of those willing to perform 'extreme sports' activity.

*Skydiving*

While risk factors and preventive measures have been addressed in civilian and military parachute jumping (fig. 2) [14, 16, 17, 23, 46–48, 56], few studies thus far have reported on prevention associated with sports jumping under more extreme conditions.

Use of a helmet, kneepads, and ankle braces may prevent injuries in airborne activities, as reported in similar sport activities [46, 48, 60–62]. An injury reduction by 40–50% as reported for preventive ankle braces worn by military paratroopers can be extrapolated to some degree to civilian skydiving [61, 63], although no direct or immediate comparison can be made.

However, since BASE jumping may be even more challenging than regular skydiving, a higher degree of vigilance and critical judgment is required in every step from the jump zone, free fall, parachute release, flying the parachute, to landing. External factors, including location, weather and wind conditions may further influence on performance. Thus, adverse events are more likely to occur.

Extrapolating evidence from military training – although both equipment and procedures may differ – demonstrates effectiveness in wearing protective ankle bracing. In fact, studies show that bruised or fractured ankles occur twice as often in those not wearing this protective gear [61, 62, 64]. In fact, simulation and test results performed for military parachute training [65] may have some extrapolated learning effects for civilian, recreational skydiving, although immediate comparison cannot be done.

## Further Research

Current availability, data details and completeness of injuries sustained in these three airborne sport events are altogether limited, scarce and heterogeneous. This severely hampers drawing firm conclusions from the current available literature. For all three sports, attempts at producing standardized report systems including incidence and prevalence numbers should be attempted.

Bungee jumping appears to suffer the most from incoherent, fragmented and case-based reports, with no structured reports or database surveillance to gather information on injury profiles. An opportunity for interested organizations should be taken towards reporting this risk-associated activity beyond case reports.

Current data on BASE jumping is limited to a few reports from Norway, Sweden and New Zealand [7–9], and one combined report on air sport injuries from Switzerland [6]. This reflects the scarce pool of reports upon which we base our current knowledge. Provided the nature of BASE jumping will still be based on local enthusiasts, the short-term outlook for a more general and wider coverage will be highly sought for. Data collection that is uniform, complete and allows for analyses would greatly enhance the knowledge base in this area for the future.

While there is a long tradition of in-depth analysis of military training and adverse events in parachuting [12, 14, 46, 48, 61, 65–68], a direct comparison to civilian training, equipment, and hazards is difficult at best. Thus, civilian activities would need to make their own information pool from which to derive first-hand knowledge for future research. Many of the studies published on civilian/recreational/sports parachuting are dated, [4, 44, 47, 69] and only a few series report on data from the last decade [2, 21, 23, 54, 56]. Injury reporting is not standardized. For future research, injury severity should be reported by standard measures such as the Abbreviated Injury Score (AIS) [70], the Injury Severity Score (ISS), or the New Injury Severity Score (NISS) [71, 72].

The Swedish Parachute Association (SFF) national registry of skydiving injuries is one of the few trauma databases available for research on sport parachuting. However, a point-prevalence survey demonstrated low sensitivity in data reporting (from 0.37 to 0.61) which in turn would yield false low-incidence calculations [73]. Attitudes to reporting may be of value to study, to understand the drivers and constraints for achieving a more complete notification of skydiving injuries.

The current reporting or collection of incident data appears random and not uniform across studies for bungee jumping and BASE jumping, while somewhat less so for skydiving. Future reports should aim to provide a uniform consensus reporting for both analysis of the event itself, the risk factors associated with the event as well as the consequences in terms of physical harm, both in the short and long term.

## References


1 Pain MT, Pain MA: Essay: risk taking in sport. Lancet 2005;366(suppl 1):S33–S34.

2 Westman A, Bjornstig U: Fatalities in Swedish skydiving. Accid Anal Prev 2005;37:1040–1048.

3 Barrows TH, Mills TJ, Kassing SD: The epidemiology of skydiving injuries: World Freefall Convention, 2000–2001. J Emerg Med 2005;28:63–68.

4 Griffith JD, Hart CL: A summary of US skydiving fatalities: 1993–1999. Percept Mot Skills 2002;94: 1089–1090.

5 Ellitsgaard N: Parachuting injuries: a study of 110,000 sports jumps. Br J Sports Med 1987;21: 13–17.

6 Hasler RM, Huttner HE, Keel MJ, et al: Spinal and pelvic injuries in airborne sports: a retrospective analysis from a major Swiss trauma centre. Injury 2012;43:440–445.

7 Monasterio E, Mei-Dan O: Risk and severity of injury in a population of BASE jumpers. NZ Med J 2008;121:70–75.

8 Søreide K, Ellingsen CL, Knutson V: How dangerous is BASE jumping? An analysis of adverse events in 20,850 jumps from the Kjerag Massif, Norway. J Trauma 2007;62:1113–1117.

9 Westman A, Rosen M, Berggren P, Bjornstig U: Parachuting from fixed objects: descriptive study of 106 fatal events in BASE jumping, 1981–2006. Br J Sports Med 2008;42:431–436.

10 Field CA, Claassen CA, O'Keefe G: Association of alcohol use and other high-risk behaviors among trauma patients. J Trauma 2001;50:13–19.

11 Spain DA, Boaz PW, Davidson DJ, et al: Risk-taking behaviors among adolescent trauma patients. J Trauma 1997;43:423–426.

12 Lillywhite LP: Analysis of extrinsic factor associated with 379 injuries occurring during 34,236 military parachute descents. J R Army Med Corps 1991;137: 115–121.

13 Pirson J, Pirlot M: A study of the influence of body weight and height on military parachute landing injuries. Mil Med 1990;155:383–385.

14 Mellen PF, Sohn SS: Military parachute mishap fatalities: a retrospective study. Aviat Space Environ Med 1990;61:1149–1152.
15 Mellen PF: Parachute static line injury with vascular compromise. Mil Med 1989;154:364–365.
16 Lowdon IM, Wetherill MH: Parachuting injuries during training descents. Injury 1989;20:257–258.
17 Pirson J, Verbiest E: A study of some factors influencing military parachute landing injuries. Aviat Space Environ Med 1985;56:564–567.
18 Schlunsen C: Bungee jumping. From a test of male courage to leisure fun of the 'Dangerous Sports Club' (in German). Z Orthop Ihre Grenzgeb 1998; 136:Oa10–11.
19 Hite PR, Greene KA, Levy DI, Jackimczyk K: Injuries resulting from bungee-cord jumping. Ann Emerg Med 1993;22:1060–1063.
20 Wolf BC, Harding BE: Patterns of injury in a fatal BASE jumping accident. Am J Forensic Med Pathol 2008;29:349–351.
21 Westman A, Bjornstig U: Injuries in Swedish skydiving. Br J Sports Med 2007;41:356–364.
22 Westman A: Shoulder injuries have been noted as a recurring problem in skydiving. J Trauma 2005;59: 1033.
23 Hart CL, Griffith JD: Rise in landing-related skydiving fatalities. Percept Mot Skills 2003;97:390–392.
24 Jain AK, Gaynon M: Images in clinical medicine. Macular hemorrhage from bungee jumping. N Engl J Med 2007;357:e3.
25 Diniz JR, Arantes TE, Urbano RV, Danda DM, Almeida DD: Ocular alterations associated with bungee jumping: case report (in Portuguese). Arq Bras Oftalmol 2005;68:853–856.
26 Curtis EB, Collin HB: Ocular injury due to bungee jumping. Clin Exp Optom 1999;82:193–195.
27 Krott R, Mietz H, Krieglstein GK: Orbital emphysema as a complication of bungee jumping. Med Sci Sports Exerc 1997;29:850–852.
28 Van Rens E: Traumatic ocular haemorrhage related to bungee jumping. Br J Ophthalmol 1994;78:948.
29 Simons R, Krol J: Visual loss from bungee jumping. Lancet 1994;343:853
30 Jain BK, Talbot EM: Bungee jumping and intraocular haemorrhage. Br J Ophthalmol 1994;78:236–237.
31 Innocenti E, Bell TA: Ocular injury resulting from bungee-cord jumping. Eye (Lond) 1994;8:710–711.
32 Habib NE, Malik TY: Visual loss from bungee jumping. Lancet 1994;343:487.
33 Filipe JA, Pinto AM, Rosas V, Castro-Correia J: Retinal complications after bungee jumping. Int Ophthalmol 1994;18:359–360.
34 David DB, Mears T, Quinlan MP: Ocular complications associated with bungee jumping. Br J Ophthalmol 1994;78:234–235.
35 Chan J: Ophthalmic complications after bungee jumping. Br J Ophthalmol 1994;78:239.
36 Amgwerd MG: Acute venous stasis in the area of the head after bungee-jumping. A report of two cases (in German). Unfallchirurg 1995;98:447–448.
37 Huang KW, Huang SJ, Lin TH, Yen ZS, Chen SC: Anterior dislocation of the humeral head from bungee jumping. Am J Emerg Med 2001;19:322–324.
38 Omololu AB, Travlos J: Bungee jumping causing a comminuted proximal femoral fracture. Injury 1995;26:413–414.
39 Zhou W, Huynh TT, Kougias P, El Sayed HF, Lin PH: Traumatic carotid artery dissection caused by bungee jumping. J Vasc Surg 2007;46:1044–1046.
40 Bungee jumping; in http://en.wikipedia.org/wiki/ [accessed 20.05.2011].
41 Hennig J, Laschefski U, Opper C: Biopsychological changes after bungee jumping: β-endorphin immunoreactivity as a mediator of euphoria? Neuropsychobiology 1994;29:28–32.
42 Van Westerloo DJ, Choi G, Lowenberg EC, et al: Acute stress elicited by bungee jumping suppresses human innate immunity. Mol Med 2011;17:180–188.
43 Hasler RM, Exadaktylos AK, Bouamra O, et al: Epidemiology and predictors of spinal injury in adult major trauma patients: European cohort study. Eur Spine J 2011;20:2174–2180.
44 Ellitsgaard N, Cuadros Ellitsgaard V, Ellitsgaard C: Injury producing factors in sport parachuting. J Sports Med Phys Fitness 1989;29:405–409.
45 Chubb RM, Lentz EC, Shannon RH: Correlation of parachute landing injuries and surface wind velocity. Aerosp Med 1964;35:962–965.
46 Schmidt MD, Sulsky SI, Amoroso PJ: Effectiveness of an outside-the-boot ankle brace in reducing parachuting related ankle injuries. Inj Prev 2005;11: 163–168.
47 Dawson M, Asghar M, Pryke S, Slater N: Civilian parachute injuries; 10 years on and no lessons learned. Injury 1998;29:573–575.
48 Amoroso PJ, Ryan JB, Bickley B, et al: Braced for impact: reducing military paratroopers' ankle sprains using outside-the-boot braces. J Trauma 1998;45:575–580.
49 Ellitsgaard N, Warburg F: Movements causing ankle fractures in parachuting. Br J Sports Med 1989;23: 27–29.
50 Výborný P, Bechná B, Zízalová D: Ocular complications after jumping from a bridge (bungee-jumping) (in Czech). Cesk Slov Oftalmol 1995;51:194–195.
51 Torre PR, Williams GG, Blackwell T, Davis CP: Bungee jumper's foot drop peroneal nerve palsy caused by bungee cord jumping. Ann Emerg Med 1993;22:1766–1767.

52 Manos D, Hamer O, Muller NL: Pulmonary hemorrhage resulting from bungee jumping. J Thorac Imaging 2007;22:358–359.
53 FitzGerald JJ, Bassi S, White BD: A subdural haematoma following 'reverse' bungee jumping. Br J Neurosurg 2002;16:307–308.
54 Hart CL, Griffith JD, Randell JA: An analysis of US parachuting fatalities: 2000–2004. Percept Mot Skills 2006;103:896–900.
55 BASE fatality list; in http://www.splatula.com/bfl/ [accessed on 21.05.2011].
56 Lee CT, Williams P, Hadden WA: Parachuting for charity: is it worth the money? A 5-year audit of parachute injuries in Tayside and the cost to the NHS. Injury 1999;30:283–287.
57 Vidovic M, Rugai N: Are hook turns a major obstacle to safe skydiving? A study of skydiving fatalities in the United States from 1992 to 2005. Percept Mot Skills 2007;105:795–802.
58 Vanderford L, Meyers M: Injuries and bungee jumping. Sports Med 1995;20:369–374.
59 Shapiro MJ, Marts B, Berni A, Keegan MJ: The perils of bungee jumping. J Emerg Med 1995;13:629–631.
60 Sulheim S, Holme I, Ekeland A, Bahr R: Helmet use and risk of head injuries in alpine skiers and snowboarders. JAMA 2006;295:919–924.
61 Knapik JJ, Spiess A, Swedler DI, et al: Systematic review of the parachute ankle brace: injury risk reduction and cost effectiveness. Am J Prev Med 2010;38:S182–S188.
62 Knapik JJ, Darakjy S, Swedler D, Amoroso P, Jones BH: Parachute ankle brace and extrinsic injury risk factors during parachuting. Aviat Space Environ Med 2008;79:408–415.
63 Luippold RS, Sulsky SI, Amoroso P: Effectiveness of an external ankle brace in reducing parachuting-related ankle injuries. Inj Prev 2011;17:58–61.
64 Knapik JJ, Spiess A, Swedler D, et al: Injury risk factors in parachuting and acceptability of the parachute ankle brace. Aviat Space Environ Med 2008;79:689–694.
65 Paskoff G: Parachute opening shock simulator to determine cervical injury tolerance. Aviat Space Environ Med 2003;74:95.
66 Deaton TG, Roby JL: Injury profile for airborne operations utilizing the SF-10A maneuverable parachute. J Spec Oper Med 2010;10:22–25.
67 Hughes CD, Weinrauch PC: Military static line parachute injuries in an Australian commando battalion. ANZ J Surg 2008;78:848–852.
68 Gilliam AD, House M, Kean D, Buxton N: Injuries caused by parachute risers during foreign military parachuting. Mil Med 2006;171:1057–1058.
69 Amamilo SC, Samuel AW, Hesketh KT, Moynihan FJ: A prospective study of parachute injuries in civilians. J Bone Joint Surg Br 1987;69:17–19.
70 AAAM – Association for the Advancement of Automotive Medicine: AIS version 90, update 1995.
71 Baker SP, O'Neill B, Haddon W Jr, Long WB: The injury severity score: a method for describing patients with multiple injuries and evaluating emergency care. J Trauma 1974;14:187–196.
72 Osler T, Baker SP, Long W: A modification of the injury severity score that both improves accuracy and simplifies scoring. J Trauma 1997;43:922–926.
73 Westman A, Sjoling M, Lindberg A, Bjornstig U: The SkyNet data: demography and injury reporting in Swedish skydiving. Accid Anal Prev 2010;42: 778–783.

Prof. Kjetil Søreide, MD, PhD
Department of Surgery, Stavanger University Hospital
Stavanger Trauma Registry, POB 8100
Armauer Hansens vei 20, NO–4068 Stavanger (Norway)
Tel. +47 5151 8330, E-Mail ksoreide@mac.com

Heggie TW, Caine DJ (eds): Epidemiology of Injury in Adventure and Extreme Sports.
Med Sport Sci. Basel, Karger, 2012, vol 58, pp 130–141

# The Epidemiology of Extreme Hiking Injuries in Volcanic Environments

Travis W. Heggie[a,b] · Tracey M. Heggie[a]

[a]Bowling Green State University, Division of Sport Management, Recreation, and Tourism, Bowling Green, Ohio, USA, and [b]James Cook University, School of Public Health, Tropical Medicine and Rehabilitation Sciences, Townsville, Qld., Australia

**Abstract**

The objective of this review was to summarize the epidemiological literature for extreme hikers in volcanic environments and describe the incidence, nature and severity of injuries, the factors contributing to the injuries, and strategies for preventing injuries. Due to the relative newness of extreme hiking in volcanic environments, there are only a small handful of studies addressing the topic. Moreover, these studies are primarily focused on extreme hikers in Hawaii Volcanoes National Park. These studies found that the majority of extreme hikers in volcanic environments are inexperienced and unfamiliar with the potential hazards present in volcanic environments. The studies found that upper respiratory irritation resulting from exposure to volcanic gases and dehydration and scrapes, abrasions, lacerations, and thermal burns to the extremities were common injuries. The severity of the injuries ranged from simple on-site treat-and-release incidents to more severe incidents and even death. This review reveals a need for well-designed epidemiologic research from volcanic destinations outside of Hawaii that identify the nature and severity of injuries along with the factors contributing to injury incidents. There is also a demonstrated need for studies identifying preventive measures that reduce both the occurrence and severity of extreme hiking incidents in volcanic environments.


While there is no consensus definition of adventure or extreme sports, a growing commercial market exists for those individuals wishing to participate in a range of what are perceived as risk-taking outdoor sport activities [1]. These activities encompass the risk of traumatic injury along with illness from exposure to adverse environmental conditions. In addition, they often take place in remote destinations with little or no access to immediate medical care [2, 3]. Even if medical care is available, it usually faces challenges related to longer response and transport times, access to fewer resources, limited provider experience due to lower patient volumes, and more extreme geographic and environmental challenges [4].

Hiking, also known as trekking, tramping, and bushwalking is a popular outdoor sport activity. In the USA alone, hiking has been one of the fastest growing outdoor sport activities since the end of World War II with a reported participation of approximately 30 million hikers [5, 6]. In many regions of the world, hiking is considered a form of exercise that helps maintain a healthy lifestyle [7]. For example, whether hiking long or short distances, hiking is considered a continuous low-intensity form of exercise that has positive effects on the human cardiovascular and cardiopulmonary systems in addition to the active and passive structures of the locomotor system [7, 8]. In other regions of the world, hiking is increasingly viewed as an extreme sport activity and a much more intense experience. While some may question whether hiking should be considered an extreme sport, it is important to recognize that expanding road, rail, and air networks in cooperation with operations such as mechanized mountain lifts and improved equipment have made more and more remote and extreme destinations accessible to hikers [9, 10].

One example of extreme hiking is that taking place in volcanic environments. Despite the potential risk to human life, active volcanoes have become popular attractions for extreme hikers seeking the ultimate intensive adventure [11]. With over 1,500 active volcanoes worldwide, extreme hiking ventures to the unpredictable and potentially hostile phenomena present at volcanoes such as those in Japan, Italy, Iceland, New Zealand, and Hawaii has increased [12, 13]. In the USA alone, over 8 million people per year visit national parks with volcanic resources each year [12]. Likewise, national parks and other protected areas worldwide such as Arenal Volcano National Park in Costa Rica, Etna Provincial Park in Italy, Vesuvius National Park in Italy, and Fuji-Hakone-Izu National Park in Japan report over 109 million visitors each year [12].

One of the most sought-after attractions for extreme hikers in volcanic environments is the opportunity to observe active lava flows and other volcanic activity such as eruptions from close proximity [12]. This makes it especially important for hikers to recognize that extreme hiking in volcanic environments entails a degree of risk that is constantly changing and difficult to remove. Furthermore, as more extreme hikers visit volcanic environments, it is almost inevitable that there will be an increase of traumatic incidents involving these hikers [14–16]. This review summarizes the epidemiological literature on extreme hiking injuries in volcanic environments and describes the nature and severity of these incidents, the factors contributing to these incidents, and the potential efficacy of any preventive strategies. For the purpose of this review, injuries are defined as any physical injury or illness incurred as a result of hiking in volcanic environments. PubMed, Medline, ProQuest International, Science Direct, Academic Search Premier, and Google Scholar were searched and all publications were assessed for their relevance to this review. A major limitation of the research reviewed is a paucity of literature on the topic. Whereas a sizeable literature addressing volcanic hazards, disaster response, and threats to surrounding communities exists, only a handful of studies addressing the relatively young activity of extreme hiking in volcanic environments exist [11, 13, 15].

## Who Is Affected by Injury?

Volcanic environments differ from usual conditions in at least one of the following variables of the physical environment: (1) the breathing atmosphere, which consists of gas composition, barometric pressure, humidity, and temperature; (2) the body envelope, which includes anything in physical contact with the subject such as lava, ambient pressure, clothing, air or water temperature, and humidity, and (3) radiation from energy sources such as heat or emissions [17].

This type of environment is not selective amongst extreme hikers and therefore makes identifying any demographic characteristic more prone to injury extremely difficult. If anything, any demographic characteristic is likely more a function of the participant make up. For example, in a 2004 case series study of 804 extreme hiker injuries and illnesses reported in Hawaii Volcanoes National Park, 63% of all hikers were male compared to 37% female and ranged from 7 to 89 years of age [15]. More telling is the fact that out the 804 extreme hikers attempting to hike to active lava flows, less than 10% were from Hawaii and over 90% were foreign nationals largely unfamiliar with volcanic environments [15]. Table 1 shows that the majority of the extreme hikers were from the mainland USA, Europe, and Asia. Given the remoteness of many volcanoes from major population centers, it is likely that the participant demographic of extreme hiking on volcanoes will consist of a strong international character.

## Where Does Injury Occur?

### *Anatomical Location*

Understanding the nature of volcanic environments is the key to understanding the anatomical location of injuries and the type of illnesses incurred by extreme hikers. For example, hiking on volcanic terrain can be tough on shoes and hiking boots. The terrain is uneven and rugged at almost every step and the younger the substrate, the more difficult the hike. In addition, younger substrates typically consist of rugged and uneven basaltic terrain with a thin layer of silica on the surface. Falls on this substrate are not only potentially jarring to bones but are also similar to falls on glass. In the 2004 study of injuries and illnesses incurred by 804 extreme hikers in Hawaii Volcanoes National Park, the authors found that 59% of the hikers sustained scrapes and abrasions to their hands, arms, legs, and head, and 51% of the hikers developed blisters on their feet [15]. Only 5% of the hikers received thermal burns from lava or hot water near the point where lava enters the Pacific Ocean. Lower extremity regions such as the feet, ankles, and knees accounted for most of the injuries followed by axial head injuries and upper extremity injuries to the arms, elbows, hands, and wrist [15].

**Table 1.** Island, state or country of residence reported by lava hikers (n = 804) (source: Heggie and Heggie [15])

| | Number | Total % of study population |
|---|---|---|
| North America | | |
| California | 137 | 17 |
| Texas | 52 | 6 |
| New York | 31 | 4 |
| Illinois | 29 | 4 |
| New Jersey | 28 | 3 |
| Florida | 25 | 3 |
| Colorado | 21 | 3 |
| Other | 184 | 23 |
| Subtotal | 507 | 63 |
| Europe | | |
| Germany | 39 | 5 |
| England | 32 | 4 |
| Switzerland | 17 | 2 |
| Austria | 15 | 2 |
| Netherlands | 10 | 1 |
| Poland | 8 | 1 |
| Subtotal | 121 | 15 |
| Asia | | |
| Japan | 62 | 8 |
| South Korea | 10 | 1 |
| Taiwan | 5 | <1 |
| Hong Kong | 3 | <1 |
| Subtotal | 80 | 10 |
| Hawaii | | |
| Oahu | 46 | 6 |
| Hawaii | 19 | 2 |
| Maui | 5 | 1 |
| Kauai | 1 | <1 |
| Molokai | 1 | <1 |
| Subtotal | 72 | 9 |
| Other | | |
| Australia | 8 | 1 |
| New Zealand | 8 | 1 |
| Israel | 6 | 1 |
| Brazil | 2 | <1 |
| Subtotal | 24 | 3 |

**Table 2.** Potential hazards threatening extreme hikers in volcanic environments (source: Hansell et al. [18], adapted from table 1)

| Hazard | Potential health effects |
|---|---|
| Acid rain | Irritant to eyes and skin. Also a potential threat to safe drinking water. Forms when rain falls through volcanic gas and acid particle emissions. Also forms where lava enters ocean water. |
| Earthquakes | Impact injuries from damage to tourist facilities and other structures. Earthquakes are common with volcanic activity. A tsunami may occur if water is displaced by underwater volcanoes. |
| Lava flows | Thermal injuries. Methane explosions can occur as active lava flows over vegetation. Lacerations, scrapes and abrasions, muscle strains and sprains, and other fall injuries when inactive lava flows used for recreational purposes. |
| Landslides/ mudflows | Burial, drowning, and impact injuries. May create a localized tsunami if either flow into an ocean or lake. |
| Laze | Irritant to eyes, skin, mucous membranes, and throat. Exposure to high concentrations can cause laryngeal spasms and pulmonary edema. |
| Pyroclastic density | Thermal and impact injuries. Forms when a mixture of hot currents ash, rocks, and gas is pulled down a volcano by gravity. |
| Tephra and ash | Impact injuries, skin and eye abrasions, and respiratory irritation. Long-term exposure can result in silicosis and chronic obstructive pulmonary disease. Hazardous to aircraft and the structural capability of facilities. Lightning is common in ash clouds. |
| Volcanic gases | Asphyxiation, vomiting, headache, dizziness, visual disturbances, tachycardia, respiratory irritation, bronchitis, bronchopneumonia, eye irritation and throat irritation. |

*Environmental Location*

Table 2 displays a list of potential hazards facing extreme hikers in volcanic environments [18]. One of the least recognized hazards facing extreme hikers in volcanic environments is that of volcanic gases. Gases such as carbon dioxide ($CO_2$), sulfur dioxide ($SO_{2)}$, hydrogen chloride (HCl), hydrogen sulfide ($H_2S$), hydrogen fluoride (HF), carbon monoxide (CO), nitrogen ($N_2$), hydrogen ($H_2$), helium (He), methane ($CH_4$) and radon (Rn) are common in volcanic environments during and in between eruptions [19, 20]. For the unsuspecting hiker, exposure to various concentrations of the odorless $CO_2$ gas can create problems ranging from vomiting and headaches to unconsciousness and the risk of asphyxiation [19]. Because $CO_2$ is denser than air, it can even pose problems for extreme hikers along low-lying hiking trails and thermal areas [19]. Likewise, exposure to various concentrations of $H_2S$ can result in upper respiratory irritation and bronchopneumonia and $SO_2$ can be an irritant to the eyes, throat, and respiratory tract [19] $SO_2$ can also pose health challenges to extreme hikers with preexisting asthmatic conditions [21]. In the previously mentioned 2004 study of injuries and illnesses incurred by 804 extreme hikers in Hawaii Volcanoes National Park, 77% reported suffering dehydration, 46% reported respiratory irritation resulting from exposure to volcanic gases, 13% reported eye irritations due to exposure to high winds and volcanic fumes, 4% experienced asthma attacks, 3% suffered from heat stroke, and 3 individuals went into cardiac distress [15].

### When Does Injury Occur?

Due to the relative newness of extreme hiking in volcanic environments and the fact that only a few studies addressing injuries incurred by these hikers actually exist, any information related to the onset of injuries and the chronometry of injuries is non-existent. Injuries such as broken bones, thermal burns from contact with lava, scrapes, abrasions, and lacerations incurred after falls onto volcanic substrates can be expected to be acute injuries. Other injuries such as blisters and muscle strains and sprains can gradually develop over time. Likewise, incidents involving dehydration and heat stroke develop over time whereas respiratory irritation resulting from exposure to volcanic gases is almost immediate depending on the concentration of the gases.

### What Is the Outcome?

Due to the varying degrees of potential danger existing in volcanic environments, the type of injuries incurred by extreme hikers can range from minor scrapes and abrasions to more severe respiratory irritation cases. For example, in the Hawaii Volcanoes National Park study, 6% suffered broken bones from falling on the substrate, 3% suffered dislocations, 47% suffered muscle strains and sprains, and 27% sustained lacerations after falling on the substrate [15]. The severity of the injuries can range from simple on-site treat-and-release incidents to more severe incidents and even death. Table 3 provides examples of the type and severity of some injuries reported in Hawaii Volcanoes National Park between 1992 and 2002 [22]. For example, the hiking incident reported in February 1993 resulted in minor scrapes and abrasions and dehydration whereas the hiking incidents reported in November 2000 and October 2002 resulted in severe respiratory irritation and the eventual death of the hikers. Table 4 provides a detailed case report of the November 2000 incident that resulted in the death of two hikers. This incident highlights the potential severe conditions present when hiking in volcanic environments where lava flows into seawater.

### What Are the Risk Factors?

Few risk factors involving extreme hikers in volcanic areas have been tested for correlation or for predictive value. It is recognized that people often underestimate the

**Table 3.** Summary of fatal and non-fatal extreme hiker injuries in Hawaii Volcanoes National Park, 1992–2002 (source: Heggie [22], adapted from table 1)

| Date reported | Description of the incident |
|---|---|
| 02/93 | A hiker became lost and suffered minor scrapes and abrasions and dehydration while hiking 5 km to active lava flows at night. The hiker did not carry drinking water or a flashlight. Search and rescue operations cost USD 4,000. |
| 04/93 | A Vietnamese national died and 16 other hikers were injured when a coastal land bench on which they were standing to view lava entering the ocean collapsed. The hikers ignored warning signs in the area. |
| 05/93 | A Japanese tourist died after falling into an active lava tube. |
| 06/93 | A 43-year-old male teacher collapsed and died from a heart attack while guiding and hiking with high school students to active lava flows. Dense volcanic fumes were measured in the area at the time of the incident. |
| 06/93 | A hiker with asthma died from a severe asthma attack after exposure to sulfur-based fumes. |
| 06/93 | A hiker died from a fatal 200 m fall into Kilauea Caldera. |
| 06/94 | A 28-year-old American female died after falling into Halemaumau Crater. |
| 07/94 | A 38-year-old American male from California sustained second-degree burns to his left leg when a wave of lava heated water washed ashore. The hiker had ignored warning signs and was standing only 4 m from the ocean while attempting to view lava entering the water. |
| 08/94 | Two American hikers from California sustained second-degree burns to their chest, arms, and legs when a wave of lava heated water washed ashore. Both men were standing on a coastal bench and had ventured beyond warning signs. |
| 01/95 | A 25-year-old German hiker sustained second-degree burns when attempting to pick up active lava with a stick. |
| 01/95 | A 61-year-old female hiker sustained second-degree burns to her hands and legs after touching active lava. The tourist indicated she could not resist the urge to reach out and touch lava even though she had read warning signs. |
| 02/95 | A 63-year-old female American hiker suffered back and neck injuries after being thrown 10 m by a methane explosion approximately 40 m in front of an active lava flow. In vegetated areas, the heat from advancing lava flows generates underground gas from the combustion of organic materials such as plant roots. |
| 02/95 | An American tourist sustained minor injuries after being thrown by a methane explosion. |
| 05/95 | Two university students became lost when hiking to active lava flows at night. The students were suffering from dehydration and exhaustion when located the next morning. |
| 08/95 | A 44-year-old American female with preexisting heart and asthma conditions died of a heart attack while hiking out of a 150 m deep volcanic crater. Exertion and dense volcanic fumes in the area were reported as contributing factors. |
| 07/96 | A 35-year-old female American hiker suffered a broken leg and multiple lacerations to both legs after falling 5 m into an earthcrack. The woman was hiking in the dark at 22:00 h. |
| 08/96 | A 27-year-old American male died from heat stroke while hiking alone near active lava flows. |

**Table 3.** Continued

| Date reported | Description of the incident |
|---|---|
| 09/97 | A 38-year-old female from Colorado collapsed from heat stroke while hiking to active lava flows. |
| 01/98 | A 51-year-old male was found suffering from exhaustion after becoming lost during a night hike to active lava flows. |
| 04/98 | A 26-year-old hiking guide and 6 others died after falling 10 m onto cooling lava. The guide was operating illegally. |
| 08/98 | Three American brothers aged 7, 9, and 18 sustained minor scrapes and abrasions while attempting to hike to active lava flows at night. |
| 04/99 | Three hikers from Canada became lost while hiking to the active Pu'u O'o Vent in bad weather. Two of the tourists sustained minor injuries after spending a night in a forest. |
| 06/99 | A 19-year-old female hiker from New York fell 30 m into an earthcrack. She was hiking at night with no flashlight, ignored warning signs, and sustained multiple scrapes, abrasions, and lacerations to her head and legs. |
| 11/00 | The bodies of 2 hikers, a 41-year-old American female and a 42-year-old American male were found 40 m from the point where active lava was flowing into the ocean. The cause of death was determined to be pulmonary edema from environmental exposure to volcanic fumes. |
| 07/01 | A 38-year-old female hiker suffered multiple lacerations to both legs when attempting to hike to active lava flows in the dark and during heavy rain. |
| 07/02 | A 67-year-old hiker was revived by park rangers with an external defibrillator (AED). The hiker had recently undergone quadruple bypass surgery and was visiting an area of the park with heavy volcanic fumes. |
| 10/02 | The body of a 45-year-old female hiker from Florida was found near active lava flows. The body had contact burns from lava but the cause of death was determined to be environmental exposure to volcanic fumes. The hiker had a preexisting heart condition. |

potential dangers and overestimate their own abilities [23]. The perceived risk and the calculation of what is an acceptable risk by the individual extreme hiker is a core factor to consider in any preventive strategy. Research by the author has shown that extreme hikers in volcanic environments seem to rely on their personal judgment when they consider the potential risk of hiking into volcanic areas [23]. Often they are lacking the basic knowledge of the true conditions in volcanic environments, in their ignorance causing danger to themselves as well as possibly to others. This in turn can lead to costly rescue and recovery situations even without the contribution of volcanic activity [23].

In the Hawaii Volcanoes National Park study of extreme hiker injuries and illnesses, 52% of the extreme hikers considered themselves beginning hikers with no previous experience in volcanic environments [15]. In fact, only 12% of the 804 hikers reported having previous experience on volcanic terrain of any type in locations such as Japan,

**Table 4.** Report on the death of 2 extreme hikers in Hawaii Volcanoes National Park, November 2000 (source: adapted from Heggie et al. [11])

In November, 2000, authorities at Hawaii Volcanoes National Park received a report of 2 dead bodies found near the ocean entry in an area of the park referred to as the Eruption Site. Both bodies (1 Caucasian male, 1 Caucasian female) were approximately 91 m directly inland from the ocean entry and located on the eastern side of active lava flows. The bodies were located approximately 12 m apart from each other. In addition, the male victim had a backpack that was found 6 m west of his body. An expert geologist at the scene reported seeing no sign of volcanic spatter and no evidence of a recent explosion in the area.

The bodies were removed via a sling load attached to a Hawaii County rescue helicopter. Two days later, autopsies of the victims were conducted by a medical examiner for the County of Honolulu. Dental records identified the victims as a 43-year-old male and a 42-year-old female. Examination of the female victim found no obvious burns on her clothing. However, her state of decomposition was extremely advanced for the estimated time of death (maximum 48 h prior to body recovery) and in comparison to the male victim. According to the medical examiner, the female had perimortem first- and second-degree burns to her head, neck, shoulders, upper chest area, and to all limbs. She also had perimortem wounds to the head, face, and limbs that were superficial in nature. Examination of the male victim also found no obvious burns to his clothing. Abrasions and lacerations to his body were also perimortem and superficial in nature. There were, however, very obvious perimortem first- and second-degree burns to the his head, neck, limbs, and areas of his trunk.

During the autopsies, no evidence suggesting that lightning or violence were factors in the deaths was found. The medical examiner did report, however, that the burns were consistent with that caused by a hot gas or vapor rather than contact with hot liquid, contact with a hot object, or radiant heat. This was based on the findings of undamaged clothing and the regions of the bodies that were burnt. For example, both victims sustained burns to areas that were unprotected or protected by a single layer of clothing. No burns were indicated or obvious where there were three layers of clothing. In areas where there were two layers of clothing there were some burns indicated and observed where the clothing may have been penetrated or tucked up. The final cause of death determined by the medical examiner was death as a result of pulmonary edema caused by inhalation of volcanic laze sustained when they were exposed to the plume near the ocean entry.

This incident highlights a potential hazard when entering areas of volcanic activity. What makes this a case of interest is that it was the first known incident of its nature in Hawaii and that it specifically highlights a potential global hazard present in locations where lava enters ocean waters. Conditions near the ocean entry typically involve exposure to volcanic laze, a dense hydrochloric acid mist that is formed when hot lava enters the ocean. This laze is often mistakenly referred to as a steam plume. Heat from the lava entering the ocean rapidly boils and vaporizes seawater producing a large white plume. This plume contains a mixture of hydrochloric acid (HCl) and concentrated seawater that is a brine with a salinity about 2.3 times that of seawater and a pH of 1.5–2.0. Moreover, dense laze plumes are known to contain as much as 10–15 ppm of HCl. These values drop off as the plume moves away from the ocean entry but acid rain commonly precipitates on individuals and land near its proximity. Hence, following the inhalation of the laze, the bodies of the victims were exposed to extreme heat and acidic conditions during the maximum 48 h they were at the ocean entry. This explains the advanced stage of decomposition of the female body which was the closest body to the ocean entry.

In addition to the cost of life, the final cost of this incident included USD 3,025 for aircraft assistance and USD 9,507 for personnel costs.

Italy, Indonesia, and Iceland [15]. Those considered beginning hikers in this study were found to be significantly more vulnerable to injury than the more experienced hikers [15]. Of further concern was the willingness of 63% of the extreme hikers to ignore posted warning signs and hike into areas exposing themselves to immediate and exceptionally dangerous conditions. In fact, only 24% of the extreme hikers took the time to read warning and information signs posted at the entrance points of active volcanic areas or speak with park authorities prior to beginning their hike.

Additional risk factors in the study from Hawaii Volcanoes National Park deal with the preparedness and preexisting health status of the extreme hikers. For example, 73% of the extreme hikers carried less than 1 liter of water with them, an amount that is below the recommended amount of water required per person. Furthermore, only 14% of the extreme hikers wore adequate hiking boots capable of withstanding a rugged basaltic terrain whereas 57% wore a version of running shoes that could tear easily on the terrain and burn easy when near active lava flows [15]. Only 3% wore protective gloves to protect their hands from cuts and abrasions when falling and only 16% carried extra batteries for their flashlights. In terms of preexisting health conditions, 37% of the extreme hikers indicated they were suffering from traveler's diarrhea prior to beginning their hike, 22% reported that they were asthmatic, 29% reported having cardiac concerns, 4% reported being pregnant, and 5% were intoxicated at the time they started their extreme hike [15].

## Injury Prevention

To date there are no known studies which have tested the effectiveness of preventive measures for extreme hikers in volcanic environments. However, there are a few practical suggestions based on the experience of park managers at Hawaii Volcanoes National Park that, when applied in other locations, may prove successful to preventing injuries to extreme hikers.

Despite their goal of facilitating safe public access to active volcanism, in 2000 managers at Hawaii Volcanoes National Park realized they faced three specific safety challenges [23]. First, lava flows and other volcanic activity in the park are dynamic and constantly changing. Second, volcanic activity and the opportunity to hike to active lava flows are heavily marketed by a variety of non-park sources. Third, after arriving on the island, extreme hikers and other tourists receive misinformation from locals and others employed in the hospitality and lodging industry. An example of such misinformation was the encouragement to hike to the active lava flows at night even though there are no marked trails.

To counter these challenges, park managers adopted a risk management strategy adapted from the Continuum of Travel Medicine [24]. Park managers developed a more informative website with the objective of providing valuable safety information to extreme hikers before they began their trip to Hawaii. Park managers then developed an 'Eruption Update' telephone hotline to combat misinformation received once the hikers arrived on island. Park managers collaborated with hospitality and lodging facilities in Hawaii to provide the number of the hotline to potential hikers. When called, the hotline provided up to the hour information on volcanic conditions in the park and also reminded hikers of maximum safety initiatives such as wearing adequate footwear, carrying the right amount of water, and the benefit of hiking during daylight hours. Finally, when extreme hikers entered the park they were reminded of safety issues in the park visitor center and a video/CD at the actual eruption site that played safety messages every few minutes. The park managers believe that these preventive methods have reduced the incidence and severity of injury in the park, however this difference has not yet been verified statistically.

## Future Research

Due to the fact that extreme hiking in volcanic environments is a relatively young activity, there is a need for a wide variety of future research initiatives. For example, more research into the motives of extreme hikers in volcanic environments is needed. It is obvious from this review that many of the extreme hikers are lacking in experience and are making decisions regarding when they themselves are not aware of all the hazards present in volcanic environments. Hence, they are beginning their extreme hike without the best of equipment and supplies, without a clear understanding of the hazards present in volcanic environments, and without caution for their preexisting health conditions. As previously noted, individuals such as the extreme hikers are known to often underestimate the potential dangers and overestimate their own abilities [23]. Thus, the perceived risk and the calculation of what is an acceptable risk by the extreme hikers is likely a core factor to consider in any preventive strategy.

A further future need is the collection of information on the epidemiology of injuries to extreme hikers in volcanic environments and the contributing factors outside of Hawaii as well as the collection of information on successful injury prevention strategies. These could include modifiable strategies on the part of extreme hikers or any government or regulatory body that may be overseeing the activity. Locations such as Mount Etna in Italy, Cerro Negro in Nicaragua, Mount Nyamulagira in the Democratic Republic of Congo, Mount Yasur volcano in Vanuatu, and multiple volcanic destinations in Guatemala and Iceland are some of the fastest growing popular destinations for extreme hikers. Any data examining the epidemiology of injuries to extreme hikers in these volcanic environments would further help identify any trends and contributing factors that in turn will assist the development of preventive measures.

## References


1 Heggie TW, Jorgenson JD: Two deaths in two days: a case report of mountaineering fatalities on Mount Rainier. Med Sport 2010;14:24–27.

2 Zell SC: Environmental and recreational hazards associated with adventure travel. J Travel Med 1997; 4:94–99.

3 Heggie TW, Heggie TM, Kliewer C: Recreational travel fatalities in US National Parks. J Travel Med 2008;15:404–411.

4 Heggie TW, Heggie TM: Saving tourists: the status of emergency medical services in California's National Parks. Travel Med Infect Dis 2009;7:19–24.

5 Boulware DR, Forgey WW, Martin WJ: Medical risks of wilderness hiking. Am J Med 2003;114: 288–293.

6 Howatson G, Hough P, Pattison J, Hill JA, Blagrove R, Glaister M, Thompson KG: Trekking poles reduce exercise-induced muscle injury during mountain walking. Med Sci Sport Exerc 2011;43: 140–145.

7 Bohne M, Abendroth-Smith J: Effects of hiking downhill using trekking poles while carrying external loads. Med Sci Sport Exerc 2007;39:177–183.

8 Schwameder H, Roithner R, Muller E, Niessen W, Raschner C: Comparison of lower extremity joint kinetics during downhill walking with and without hiking poles. J Sport Sci 1999;17:969–968.

9 Mieske K, Flaherty G, O'Brien T: Journeys to high altitude: risks and recommendations for travelers with preexisting medical conditions. J Travel Med 2010;17:48–62.

10 Heggie TW: Paediatric and adolescent sport injury in the wilderness. Br J Sports Med 2010;44:50–55.

11 Heggie TW, Heggie TM, Heggie TJ: Death by volcanic laze. Wilderness Environ Med 2009;20: 101–103.

12 Erfurt-Cooper P, Cooper M: An introduction to volcano and geothermal tourism; in Erfurt-Cooper P, Cooper M (eds): Volcano and Geothermal Tourism: sustainable Geo-Resources for leisure and Recreation. Washington, Earthscan, 2010, pp 3–31.

13 Heggie TW, Kupper T, Heggie TM: Spezifische Gefahren bei Vulkan-Tourismus. Arbeitsmed Sozialmed Umwelt 2010;45:678–683.

14 Benediktsson K, Anna Lund K, Huijbens E: Inspired by eruptions? Eyjafjallajökull and Icelandic tourism. Mobilities 2011;6:77–84.

15 Heggie TW, Heggie TM: Viewing lava safely: an epidemiology of hiker injury and illness in Hawaii Volcanoes National Park. Wilderness Environ Med 2004;15:77–81.

16 Thór Jóhannessona G, Edward H: Tourism in times of crisis: exploring the discourse of tourism development in Iceland. Curr Issues Tourism 2010;13: 419–434.

17 Dillard TA, Khosla S, Ewald FW, Asif Kaleem M: Pulmonary function testing in extreme environments. Clin Chest Med 2005;26:485–507.

18 Hansell AL, Horwell CJ, Oppenheimer C: Health hazards of volcanoes and geothermal areas. Occup Environ Med 2006;63:149–156.

19 Heggie TW: Geotourism and volcanoes: health hazards facing tourists at volcanic and geothermal destinations. Travel Med Infect Dis 2009;7:257–261.

20 Cantrell L, Young M: Fatal fall into a volcanic fumarole. Wilderness Environ Med 2009;20:77–79.

21 Heggie TW: Volcanoes and travel medicine. Travel Med Infect Dis 2010;8:199–200.

22 Heggie TW: Reported fatal and non-fatal incident involving tourists in Hawaii Volcanoes National Park, 1992–2002. Travel Med Infect Dis 2005;3: 123–131.

23 Erfurt-Cooper P, Heggie TW: Risk Perception, Prevention, Management and Mitigation in Volcanic Environments. Proceedings of the Inaugural Global Geotourism Conference, Perth, Australia, 2008, pp 427–430.

24 Leggat PA, Ross MH, Goldsmid JM: Introduction to Travel Medicine; in Leggat PA, Goldsmid JM (eds): Primer of Travel Medicine, ed 3. Brisbane, ACTM Publications, 2005, pp 3–21.



Travis W. Heggie, PhD
Bowling Green State University
Division of Sport Management, Recreation and Tourism
210 Eppler North, Bowling Green, OH 43403 (USA)
Tel. +1 419 372 2395, E-Mail theggie@bgsu.edu

Heggie TW, Caine DJ (eds): Epidemiology of Injury in Adventure and Extreme Sports.
Med Sport Sci. Basel, Karger, 2012, vol 58, pp 142–157

# The Epidemiology of Injury in Skateboarding

Jamie Hunter

University of Manchester, Manchester, UK

**Abstract**

The purpose of this report is to review the available literature to provide an epidemiological overview of skateboarding injuries, as well as to suggest possible areas for future research. A literature search was performed with the databases of PubMed, Sport Discus, Google and Google Scholar using the search terms 'skateboard', 'skateboarding', 'injury' and 'injuries', with all articles published in refereed journals in the English language being considered. An ancestry approach was also used. Articles from non-juried journals were also infrequently included to provide anecdotal information on the sport. Comparison of study results was compromised by the diversity of different study populations and variability of injury definitions across studies. The majority of injuries affect young males although conflicting arguments arise over the issues of age and experience in relation to injury severity. Most injuries are acutely suffered, and the most commonly affected body part was the wrist and forearm, with lower leg and ankle injuries also common. The incidence was relatively high but reports on severity differed. Clear conclusions could not be drawn on environmental location and risk factors. Most injuries tend to occur from a loss of balance leading to a fall, in more recent times due to a failed trick. Research on injury prevention is not conclusive although protective equipment and skatepark use are recommended. Further research using more rigorous study designs is required to gain a clearer picture of the incidence and determinants of injury, and to identify risk factors and viable injury countermeasures. 

Skateboarding is believed to have begun sometime in the late 1940s or early 1950s when the surfing community of California was looking for an outlet to transfer their skills from the waves to the sidewalks [1]. This resulted in various wooden platforms being combined with the wheels from roller skates and eventually companies began producing boards of multiple pressed layers of wood to create something not dissimilar to modern-day skateboard decks. As several surfing companies started to manufacture skateboards, the popularity of this pastime grew and *Skateboarder Magazine* was first published in 1964 [2]. However, due to health and safety fears which caused many American cities to ban skateboarding, the sport had all but disappeared by the end of 1965 and after only four issues the magazine ceased publication.

The resurrection of skateboarding in the early 1970s can be attributed to the polyurethane wheel, invented by Frank Nasworthy [1]. Previous wheels made from clay or steel lacked the necessary performance that skaters' skills demanded, and this improved standard allowed the skateboarder a greater degree of control. The popularity of skateboarding increased as the technology progressed which brought about a greater range of tricks that could be performed. With faster speeds and more dangerous tricks came a high price and spiralling insurance costs forced many skateparks to close, leaving enthusiasts without a regular place to skate and forcing them to use unsuitable public or even private property. The general public and lawmakers viewed this practice as dangerous and banned skateboarding in many areas; by the 1980s the sport again slipped back into obscurity.

The last 20 years has seen an explosion in both the popularity and the participation of adventure and extreme sports, fuelled by the interest and disposable income of the current generation [3]. Skateboarding has been at the forefront of these activities with increased exposure in popular culture through television, music, fashion, video games and the internet; the resulting increase in financial backing has transformed the amateur exhibitionist into a full-time professional athlete and multimillionaire. Household names such as Tony Hawk and Shaun White regularly compete on television, culminating in the X Games – the extreme sport equivalent of the Olympics where skateboarders take part in street, vertical and 'big air' disciplines. These events require the athlete to perform different tricks and skills using various pieces of equipment such as ramps, rails, banks, ledges and half-pipes – large semicircular ramps that allow the participant to project themselves high into the air and perform multiple tricks before landing and maintaining their momentum to the opposite side where the process can be repeated several times. Points are awarded by judges for such factors as content, variety, style, degree of difficulty and originality.

As in any highly competitive professional sport, athletes push themselves to the limit to achieve new heights and break boundaries; skateboarding is no exception. Tricks have become more and more inventive and complex with these sportsmen seemingly defying gravity with increasingly difficult maneuvers. Today's icons are extremely athletic, being able to control themselves and their board at speeds of up to 40 miles an hour, flying through the air and landing in a controlled manner. They need to have excellent balance, flexibility, strength and awareness. This puts an unprecedented demand on the professional skateboarder's body and nearly every one of them has an extensively long list of previous injuries suffered as a result of their passion.

Another characteristic that skateboarding shares with all sports is the attempt by youngsters and other amateurs to emulate those at the highest level. This can be harmless in other activities, but represents a significant risk to the inexperienced skater. With many recreational participants lacking the necessary aforementioned skills and judgement to pull off such high-risk maneuvers, as well as the availability of modern equipment and the public's accessibility to skateparks, injuries are common and can sometimes be catastrophic. These events are not a recent development; skateboarding injuries have been reported in numerous journals since the 1960s [4] with the 'perilous skateboard' inciting great debate in the *British Medical Journal* as long ago as the 1970s [5]. Despite these warnings, serious injuries are still prevalent and are often tragic; in the first 6 months of 2011 alone there were two highly publicized cases in the USA involving 16- and 17-year-old males who died as a result of major head injuries [6, 7]. Notably, neither individual was wearing a helmet at the time of their accident.

According to the National Electronic Injury Surveillance System (NEISS), conducted by the US Consumer Product Safety Commission, it is estimated that 144,416 injuries related to skateboards presented to hospital emergency departments in 2009 across the nation, with the vast majority affecting males under the age of 24 [8]. The Safe Kids organization estimates that of these injuries affecting children, just over 3,000 were of a serious nature [9]. In addition, the National Sporting Goods Association (NSGA) believes that there are nearly 8 million individuals over 7 years of age who participated in skateboarding more than once in 2010 [10]. Although there continues to be this high rate of participation and frequency of injury, as well as the catastrophic stories featured in the media, there remains a distinct shortage of recent research performed on the topic of skateboarding injuries.

Several reviews of skateboarding injuries [11, 12] and in-depth case studies [13, 14] have been published, however several limitations are apparent which creates difficulty in analyzing the subject. The most recent review on this topic was performed almost 10 years ago and was based on figures from the NEISS and the NSGA, which are estimated numbers. This study was also the first to relate skateboarding injuries to participation exposures, highlighting the shortcomings of previous reviews. Very few exposure-based, cohort studies have been conducted, with the majority of research being provided by case series. Although this research is useful for formulating hypotheses, it is impossible to use them to investigate a clear statistical association and fully identify possible risk factors. Comparison between these studies is complicated by the diversity of different study populations, with discrepancies in such aspects as age, performance level and exposure hours. This may be due to skateboarding's position as a recreational activity without a reliable structure that more traditional activities and team sports possess. There may also be a seasonal element involved, with more participants in the warmer months of summer, which few studies take into account. Also many articles focus primarily on fractures sustained from skateboarding accidents and overlook other relevant injuries such as sprains, strains, lacerations and head injuries. These limitations should be taken into account when analyzing the research, yet the reader should also acknowledge the challenges faced when collecting the relevant data.

The primary aim of this report is to address the available literature to provide an epidemiological overview of skateboarding injuries, as well as to suggest possible areas for future research and further investigation. A literature search was performed with the databases of PubMed, Sport Discus, Google and Google Scholar using the search terms 'skateboard', 'skateboarding', 'injury' and 'injuries', with all articles published in refereed journals in the English language being considered. Articles from non-juried journals were also infrequently included to provide anecdotal information on the sport. The following topic areas are addressed in this report: Who is affected by injury, where does injury occur (both anatomically and environmentally), when does injury occur, what is the outcome of injury, what are the risk factors, what are the inciting events, injury prevention and future research?

## Who Is Affected by Injury?

Skateboarding has always been viewed as an activity with a high risk of injury given its association with risk-taking and dangerous behavior, the lack of structured and supervised periods of participation and the reluctance of a mainly adolescent male population to wearing personal protective equipment. The definition of an injury from skateboarding can be a difficult concept for the academic and the statistician to grasp as many injuries, particularly those of a minor nature, may go unreported. Many articles are based upon information from hospitals or emergency departments and focus on fractures sustained during skateboarding, meaning injuries of a lesser severity that are treated in a different environment are not present in the literature. Individuals may also not present to a healthcare professional and avoid certain obstacles or maneuvers to hide an injury from their peers. Although the majority of skateboarding injuries may be acutely suffered, chronic or overuse injuries can also occur and remain absent from the available literature.

Table 1 shows a comparison of demographic data across a number of studies in skateboarding. The design for most studies is case series; however, cross-sectional and retrospective cohort designs are also included. However, few of the studies are comprehensive in their content, with very little reporting of injury rates and level of experience featured. It is clear that the vast majority of injuries are suffered by males with numerous reports presenting figures of well over 90%. Males suffer from more serious injuries due to their habits of skating outdoors, in more dangerous locations and wear less protective equipment than females [15]. Also interesting to note is that several older articles from the 1960s, 1970s and 1980s show a higher degree of female involvement; this may be down to the general trend of girls showing lower participation in sports in general throughout more recent years.

The average age of those injured shows a variation from the mid-to-late teens up to the early 20s, possibly explained by the variation of data collection from both children's hospitals and those focusing on adult medicine. Several studies conclude that injured individuals tend to be at the younger end of this scale, between 10 and 15 [13, 22], and Vaca et al. [23] report that 'fewer skatepark users in the age range 15–19 years were injured'.

**Table 1.** A comparison of injury frequency in studies of skateboard injuries

| Study (first author) | Patients n | Injuries n | Injury rate | Mean age of patients | Male proportion % | Experience level |
|---|---|---|---|---|---|---|
| *Case series* | | | | | | |
| Hawkins 1981 [16] | 49 | 50 | | 14 | 73 | 0–6 months: 52%<br>6 months–1 year: 26%<br>1+ year: 22% |
| Forsman 2001 [14] | 139 | 147 | | 16 | 95 | |
| Everett 2002 [17] | 100 | 106 | 1.11/ 1,000 people | 19 | 98 | beginner: 15%<br>intermediate: 38%<br>advanced: 36%<br>professional: 11% |
| Zalavras 2005 [13] | 187 | 191 | | 13 | 95 | |
| Vaca 2007 [18] | 95 | 97 | | 20 | 98 | |
| Lustenberger 2010 [19] | 2,270 | 2,658 | | 16.9 | 91 | |
| *Cross-sectional* | | | | | | |
| Schuman 1967 [4] | 1,984 | 494 | | range: 9–15 | 77% fractures in boys | |
| Pendergrast 1990 [20] | 94 | | | | 69 | 37% non-current users<br>27% moderate users<br>36% heavy users |
| Osberg 1998 [15] | 254 | | | 12.8 | 93 | |
| Keilani 2010 [21] | 75 | | | 22 | 97 | 8 years mean experience,<br>18 h/week mean practice |

In relation to other activities, skateboarding is a comparably safe pastime [12]. Based on figures acquired from 1998, the rate of injuries treated in emergency departments (8.9 per thousand participants) was significantly lower than those for basketball and football (21.2 and 20.7, respectively). Even when compared to other adventure sports, skateboarding compared favorably with bicycling at 11.5 and snowboarding at 11.2. However, Kyle et al. [12] also found in their review that the rate of skateboarding injuries is increasing, doubling between 1993 and 1998. In a direct comparison to roller-skating and scooter-riding, pediatric patients suffering from a skateboard-

**Table 2.** A comparison of injury by anatomical location in studies of skateboarding injury

| Study (first author) | Forearm/ wrist, % | Elbow % | Hand % | Ankle % | Foot % | Leg % | Head % |
|---|---|---|---|---|---|---|---|
| *Case series* | | | | | | | |
| Illingworth, 1978 [25] | 61 | | 11 | 8 | 5 | | 1 |
| Cass, 1990 [26] | 58.6 | 4.3 | | 4.3 | | | 12.8 |
| Schieber, 1994 [27] | 19 | 6 | 11 | 11 | | 3 | 7 |
| Finch, 1998 [28] | 54.3 upper extremity | | | 17.6 lower extremity | | | 18.4 |
| Forsman, 2001 [14] | 19 | 5 | 12 | 19 | 21 | 2 | |
| Zalavras, 2005 [13] | 48.2 | 12.6 | 5.8 | 23 | 4.2 | 3.7 | |
| *Cross-sectional* | | | | | | | |
| Keilani, 2010 [21] | 77 | 67 | | 83 | | 72 | 18 |
| *Retrospective cohort* | | | | | | | |
| Konkin, 2006 [24] | 44 extremities | | | | | | 16.3 |
| Lustenberger, 2010 [19] | 27.8 upper extremity | | | 22.4 lower extremity | | | 36.3 |

related fracture tended to be older and were more likely to be male [13]. Another article investigating severe injuries in non-motorized wheeled vehicles found that skateboarders were also more likely to be male, but were younger than cyclists and in-line skaters [24]. These observations suggest that those injured in skateboarding tend to be adolescent males.

## Where Does Injury Occur?

### *Anatomical Location*

Knowledge of the anatomical location of injury can be vital for sports medicine staff as well as epidemiologists, helping to highlight which areas are more likely to be injured and assist in the direction of future preventive research. Table 2 shows skateboarding injuries by anatomical location across a selected range of articles. Not all studies of skateboarding injuries report injury by anatomical location or in a way that makes it possible to fit them into table 2. Indeed several papers purely focus on fractures suffered during skateboarding and do not cover other major injuries such as those to the internal organs or the brain, or minor injuries such as sprains and contusions.

As shown in table 2, the forearm and wrist area is the most commonly injured region of the body with several studies reporting proportions of 50% or greater. There was a discrepancy in data collection that meant only the forearm or wrist was recorded in some articles, and in others was merely referred to as 'upper extremity'. The second most frequently injured body part is the ankle (4.3–23%), and again was interpreted in different ways; 'lower leg' and 'lower extremity' both commonly used terms. Head injuries, as well as those to the neck and face, were the next most common site of injury and often produced a more severe outcome for the patient. Injuries to the elbow, foot, hand and leg were also frequently yet inconsistently reported and support the idea that musculoskeletal injuries are the most common finding in an injured skateboarder.

A review of injuries in skateboarding by Fountain and Meyers [11] supports the theory that upper extremity injuries are the most frequent, due to the participant falling on an outstretched arm. It is also reported that fractures of the upper and lower extremity account for 50% of all injuries seen in skateboarding. A second review [12] came to similar conclusions.

The high figures quoted by Keilani et al. [21] can be attributed to the study design, as all participants were active skateboarders. Skateboards reach high speeds, lack a mechanical braking system and individuals perform more complex stunts and tricks as they become more experienced, making the likelihood of an injury at any point very high.

*Environmental Location*

Very few papers have investigated the environmental location of skateboarding injuries, with mostly anecdotal evidence taking the place of reliable, structured research. Skateparks are built to provide skaters with an environment containing obstacles expressly designed for skateboarding free from traffic for their own safety, and to leave pavements and other public areas in the pedestrian's domain. In their review of NEISS data, Kyle et al. [12] found that those requiring hospitalization were 11.4 times more likely to have been injured by a motor vehicle than those who were discharged from hospital on the same day. On the other hand, Sheehan et al. [29] reported that skateparks had a relative risk of 8.35 for fractures requiring manipulation or an invasive treatment when compared to injuries suffered in the street.

The purpose of skateparks is to provide a safe and supervised area for skaters away from the dangers of traffic. Despite this, many subjects choose to skate on roads and in public places. Forsman and Eriksson [14] report that most injuries took place in specially designed areas for skateboarding, although a high frequency of injury would be expected as the same skills are being performed on similar equipment to that outside a skatepark. Another paper found that the type of terrain was not significant with respect to injury [21] whereas in a review hospitalization was 11.4 times more likely after a skateboarder experiences a crash with a motor vehicle [12].

In one article that investigated the influence of skatepark design on injuries, more incidents occurred in the ramps and bars region compared to the half-pipe and gully areas [17]. It is suggested that this may be because the ramps and bars are the most popular attractions to the skatepark users, as well as their popularization in professional competitions featured on television.

Understandably several hospitals report an increase in the frequency of skateboarding injuries when a skatepark has opened nearby [18, 30]. However, the Committee on Injury and Poison Prevention recommends that skateboards should 'never' be ridden in or near traffic and 'skitching a ride', where a skater holds onto a vehicle to gain momentum, should not be practiced [31]. Communities are also encouraged to continue developing skateparks and skateboarders to utilize these in preference to homemade jumps or ramps as they are also more easily monitored for safety.

## When Does Injury Occur?

### *Injury Onset*

In a sport such as skateboarding, where complicated tricks are conducted at high velocities on extremely hard surfaces with high-risk skills being performed, it is inevitable that sudden-onset injuries will occur frequently. A cross-sectional observation of skateboarders in Vienna discovered that 97% of respondents reported at least one injury [21]. The vast majority of studies reporting on skateboarding injuries harness data acquired from hospital emergency departments which strictly deal with acute cases, or focus on fractures that present in the same way. There are no articles that take into account more chronic or gradual-onset injuries, making the comparison between the two groups impossible.

### *Chronometry*

It would be expected that a greater proportion of injuries would be seen from skateboarding during the spring and summer months when conditions would be more favorable to spending extended periods outside. However, very few papers acknowledge this, with one article reporting that 36 out of 50 injuries were sustained during the summer [32] and another remarking that its research period 'included the winter months when accidents were likely to be fewer' [25]. Another reasonable assumption would be that more injuries occur during the day, when skating environments are bathed in natural light. An article by Hawkins and Lyne [16] concurs by revealing that most injuries seen happened during daylight hours with only 15% being sustained after 8 p.m.

As most skateboarders are recreational practitioners there are no figures for injuries suffered in competitive environments; many well-known and professional skateboarders have a long list of previously suffered injuries although this evidence is anecdotal. Research looking into the injuries of competitive skateboarders in and out of competition would be a welcome addition to the landscape of information in skateboarding. Information on skateboarding events and competitions is freely available on the internet [33].

**Table 3.** Type of injury suffered during skateboard activity

| Study (first author) | Sprain/ strain, % | Fracture % | Laceration % | Contusion/ abrasion, % | Concussion % |
|---|---|---|---|---|---|
| *Case series* | | | | | |
| Schieber, 1994 [27] | 20 | 29 | 22 | 21 | <1 |
| Forsman, 2001 [14] | 44 | 29 | 9 | 15 | 3 |
| Vaca, 2005 [23] | 15 | 60 | 7 | | 9 (closed head injuries) |
| Lustenberger, 2010 [19] | | 50.3 | | | 11.9 |
| *Review* | | | | | |
| Kyle, 2002* [12] | 14.8 | 15.2 | 8.1 | 4.9 | 2 |

* From the ten most frequently occurring emergency department-treated skateboard-associated injuries.

## What Is the Outcome?

### *Injury Type*

The various types of injury are categorized slightly differently from study to study, however it is possible to make clear comparisons. Table 3 shows the percent comparison across a range of studies of skateboarding injuries. It can be seen from the table that fractures (15.2–60%) are the most common type of injury, followed by sprains and strains (14.8–44%). Lacerations and contusions were also common injuries, with concussions less commonly reported. The distribution of injuries by type may not be truly reflective of the percent distribution of injury types actually experienced. Since these are injuries presented to the emergency departments of hospitals, they are likely to be more severe in nature. In reality we would expect to see a greater proportion of minor injuries that could be self-treated, such as lacerations and contusions.

The main difficulty in comparing the data across different studies was the definition of the different injury types and the grouping together of similar injuries such as strains and sprains and contusions and abrasions.

### *Injury Severity*

The severity of an injury is an important factor to consider in determining the relative safety and risk level of any activity. Although several articles report on how severe skateboarding injuries were in their research, there is a large variation in the way it is collected; some use Injury Severity Score (ISS), AIS system or merely describe severity in basic terms such as mild, moderate and severe. Konkin et al. [24] reported a mean ISS of 10.5 which compares favorably next to in-line skating (10.6) and cycling (12.7). A similar ISS of 8.6 was found in another article [19] that supports this finding. Lustenberger et al. [19] also described an overall rate of severe injuries at 16.2% (3.3% critical) which corresponds with similar results by Osberg et al. [15] (16.5%) and Vaca et al. [23] (15% serious, 58% moderate, 27% minor). Forsman and Eriksson [14] reported no severe injuries at all (30% moderate, 70% minor). These figures paint a picture which suggests skateboarding is relatively safe, however in a study of 75 skateboarders, 45% were reported as having suffered a severe injury in the last 2 years [21]. An open fracture of the forearm or radius was also 19 times more likely to be due to skateboarding than any other mechanism [13].

With some injuries being severe in nature, operative intervention and hospitalization may be required to treat the patient appropriately. As many as 42.2% of patients required surgery [19] with 68% of skatepark-related fractures being operated on [29]. Hospitalization rates have been quoted at 9% [23] with the average length of stay varying from 6 to 8 days [15, 23].

*Clinical Outcome*

Very little information is available on injury recurrence, non-participation, or the residual effects of injuries sustained by skateboarders. Catastrophic injuries, although rare, do occur and garner some interest in the media due to their nature; defined as a 'sport injury that resulted in a brain or spinal cord injury or skull or spinal fracture' by the National Centre for Catastrophic Injury Research, these injuries are always worrying.

Although there have been case reports of other serious injuries – notably a renal laceration [34] and a scroto-abdominal impalement injury [35] – only recently have quality data been published on catastrophic injuries. In a Canadian textbook on catastrophic injuries in sports and recreation, Tator [36] reported a total of 9 such injuries across a 4-year survey. Eight of these were suffered by males, with the same number affecting those aged between 11 and 20 years. One fatality occurred to a 10-year-old boy who suffered head and spine injuries. The annual catastrophic injury rate was 0.007%, a relatively low figure, however injuries of such magnitude and severity should never be underestimated.

Lustenberger et al. [19] also reported a severe traumatic brain injury frequency of 13.4%, including subdural hemorrhage (3.7%) and subarachnoid hemorrhage (2.3%).

*Economic Cost*

Lengthy stays in hospital and surgical interventions can cost patients and hospitals considerable sums of money; a Scottish study that looked at the impact of a new skatepark opening near a local hospital shows one example [30]. In the 12 weeks prior to the opening of the skatepark, 1.5% of sporting injuries were skatepark-related. Following the opening, this increased to 5.6%. With this rise in injuries came a direct rise in costs, which before was estimated at GBP 2,985 and increased by more than 5 times to GBP

16,862. Although this may seem fairly trivial given the large budgets of modern hospitals, this impact could be more serious on a grander scale and an area with a larger skateboarding community such as areas of the USA. It also hints at a greater economic cost to society in terms of loss from earnings due to long-term morbidity.

Vaca et al. [18] investigated such issues in an article investigating the economic impact of skatepark-related injuries in Southern California. Young patients missed on average 2 days of school as a result of their injuries, forcing parents to stay away from work to care for their child; this resulted in an average wage loss of USD 146. Furthermore, adults aged 26–39 who were injured missed an average of almost 17 days of work, amounting to an average of USD 3,163. This demonstrates the 'considerable risk' these injuries represent to employed individuals who potentially have much more to lose than their younger counterparts. There is even anecdotal evidence of injured patients with manual skills losing their jobs as a result of their injuries.

## What Are the Risk Factors?

For injury intervention and the implementation of preventive measures, an understanding of the relevant risk factors is of high importance. However this is challenging with skateboarding injuries as many studies do not specifically test for risk factors.

*Intrinsic Factors*

As discussed above, the vast majority of those injured when skateboarding are males. They are also more likely to suffer from a serious injury than females [15]. However, the relation between exposure-based injury rates and gender was not tested in the literature reviewed.

Reports on the risk related to age are conflicting. Many studies report that older, more experienced participants are more susceptible to severe injuries [19, 21, 23] whereas others believe that severity decreases with age [14]. Vaca et al. [23] also found that fewer users of skateparks between the ages of 15 and 19 were injured, as well as there being no association with experience. Another study has shown that experience does not correlate with severity [29] and neither did age. This relationship has also not been subjected to statistical tests using exposure-based injury rates.

Similar findings are seen with head injuries. In a study by Lustenberger et al. [19], a high frequency of traumatic brain injuries were suffered by skateboarders. The incidence of severe head injury increased significantly with age. It is hypothesized that this may be attributed to older participants travelling at greater velocities, on street surfaces and using helmets significantly less than their younger fellow skateboarders. This contrasts with the Tator study [36] where all catastrophic injuries were sustained by those younger than 20 years of age and the long-held theory that younger children are more susceptible to head injury [21] due to their high center of mass and psychomotor underdevelopment [11]. Nonetheless, young children do tend to be top heavy and this characteristic, combined with balance difficulties, may predispose them to injury [37].

There is an explanation for these differing results, none of which are incorrect. Although age and experience are two separate factors, they often go together and should be considered when evaluating skateboarding injuries. One would think the less experienced skateboarder would be more prone to injury, however experience has not been tested as a risk factor. The young may lack the physical and mental maturity, as well as the experience to exhibit the necessary level of control, putting them at a higher risk. Older skateboarders, from the age of 20 upwards, may also lack this experience as they are not regular practitioners. As seasoned skateboarders become older, and throughout their adolescent years their physical attributes change, their experience allows them to attempt more dangerous maneuvers at greater speeds. So it is possible to say that all levels of age and experience carry with them an element of risk in one way or another.

Results regarding the level of experience are small in number and often contradictory. Inexperienced skaters may be injured due to the alien nature of the sport, whereas those with years of practice tend to take more risks with difficult tricks performed at greater velocities [11]. Keilani et al. [21] appreciate this ambiguity, with Vaca et al. [23] also reporting that injury occurrence and severity are not strongly associated with experience level.

Very few papers report on the impact of socio-demographic details in skateboarding injuries. Those that did found that factors such as occupation, partner status, residence, education or insurance status had no significant impact [21, 23].

*Extrinsic Factors*

Protective equipment is an obvious method of trying to reduce injuries and nearly every article advocates the use of such items as helmets, elbow and knee pads as well as wrist protectors. Unfortunately no research has been performed looking specifically at the effect of not wearing personal protective gear and injuries. Rates on the use of protective equipment range from as low as 5% [29] to over 90% [23].

The teaching of certain skills such as how to fall properly and attempt tricks safely would be a useful lesson to the young skateboarder. However, due to its recreational and unstructured nature, skaters tend to learn from their friends or from watching professionals and very few receive any form of instruction before they start skateboarding [38].

### What Are the Inciting Events?

Injuries in skateboarding may occur for a variety of reasons. Table 4 shows the comparison of the mechanism of injury in skateboarding accidents across a selection of studies. Loss of balance (24.9–42) and irregularities encountered in the riding surface

**Table 4.** Mechanism of injury in skateboard-associated studies

| Study (first author) | Lost balance % | Failed trick % | Cornering/ swerving % | Skidding % | Surface irregularity % | Collision % |
|---|---|---|---|---|---|---|
| *Case series* | | | | | | |
| Illingworth, 1978 [25] | 24.9 | | 10.2 | 5.3 | 30.2 | 7.6 |
| Hawkins, 1981 [16] | 35.1 | | | 2.7 | 32.4 | 2.7 (object) |
| Forsman, 2001 [14] | 37.4 | 26 | | | 6.9 | |
| Rethnam, 2008 [32] | 42 | 56 | | | | 2 (vehicle) |
| *Cross-sectional* | | | | | | |
| Osberg, 1998 [15] | 73.6 (fall) | | | | | 24.8 (vehicle) |

(6.9–32.4) account for the majority of injuries. Presumably these led to falls from the skateboard, although only Osberg et al.'s [15] research reports on the frequency of injuries caused by 'falling'.

Interesting to note is the lack of figures quoted for a failed trick in the two earlier papers by Illingworth et al. [25] and Hawkins and Lyne [16]. This is possibly due to the advancement of skateboarding technology in allowing participants to attempt more advanced skills, hence accounting for the significant number of injuries caused by trick failure in more recent times.

Osberg et al.'s [15] results show that, despite warnings to the contrary and the obvious danger, skateboarders still use streets and highways as a location for their skills.

### Injury Prevention

A summary of preventive measures is provided in several reviews of injuries in skateboarding [11, 39] as well as the majority of articles suggesting ways in which injuries can be minimized or avoided. However, these reports are mostly intuitive with conclusions drawn from descriptive data; no studies have actually fully tested preventive measures. This is because factors such as equipment and skatepark use are extremely difficult to test. It would be dangerous and impractical to ask a control group of skateboarders to practice without any protective equipment at all for an extended period of time, and many users in the studies featured were wearing appropriate equipment [23]. Likewise difficulties exist in assessing the safety of skateparks as many skaters participate in several different locations, both custom-designed and public areas [21]. A case-control study design may demonstrate the effectiveness of protective equipment in preventing injuries presented to the emergency department as has been demonstrated with bicycle head and face injuries [40]. However, to date there are no published reports on this.

Wearing protective equipment cannot stop injuries from occurring but they can decrease the severity [11]. Despite this, adolescents wear less protective equipment than is recommended [41] and compliance with its use is not 100% even in skateparks where it is mandatory [17]. This could be because this kind of equipment is regarded as unfashionable and portrays the individual as inexperienced with limited skill, an important factor in a sport where the opinion of one's peers is often the only measurement of success. In a randomized controlled trial where helmets were given directly to pediatric patients in the emergency department, reported helmet use increased by 16 times when reported by a parent and 10 times when reported by the child [42] than those who received a voucher for a helmet or only verbal counselling. This displayed the importance of non-financial barriers to helmet use and that the biggest reason for not wearing a helmet was not owning one.

There have been huge efforts made to provide skateboarders with safe areas to practice without the dangers of traffic or in pedestrianized areas. Although their effectiveness is unclear [23], it is generally perceived that they help to reduce the severity of injuries and protect against head injuries [19].

There is tremendous scope to improve education efforts for skateboarders and their parents, teaching them about the dangers of the sport as well as techniques to avoid injury such as proper falling and rolling. This instruction and guidance could prove invaluable as very few skateboarders receive any instruction before they begin skating [38].

## Further Research

In reviewing a topic such as skateboarding injuries it is inevitable that shortcomings in the current data will be exposed and there is potential for further research to be developed. Some critical areas of research have been identified for skateboarding: (1) Prospective cohort research is required on injury in relation to exposure time and experience, which few studies have so far failed to address. (2) There is a need for greater standardization of data in several fields, notably injury severity, in order for clearer comparisons to be made across studies. (3) There also needs to be a transition to more etiologically-based research. (4) Observational data are needed to investigate skating safety behavior and the consequences, and gather further detail on injury mechanisms, risk factors and intervention strategies. (5) Case-control study designs should be used to examine the effectiveness of skateboarding safety equipment and the benefits of skatepark use. (6) Studies should be conducted comparing injuries from private skateparks to other parks and public places to test the effectiveness of safety guidelines. (7) Data on injuries suffered in competition, possibly by professionals, is an area that has been overlooked and which there are no figures currently published.

(8) There should be greater follow-up of patients to examine any long-term effects of their injuries, as well as investigation into any chronic or overuse injuries suffered by skateboarders. (9) Greater emphasis should be attributed to the education of participants and parents with research being more widely available and the dangers of injury discussed more frequently.

Further research needs to be all-inclusive and include a multidisciplinary team including skateboarders, guardians, instructors, manufacturers, physicians, physiotherapists and academics to be fully successful.

## References


1 Skateboarding History. Available at: http://www.skatelog.com/skateboarding/skateboarding-history.htm. Accessed 08/07/2011.

2 Skateboarding: A Brief History. Available at: http://skateboard.about.com/cs/boardscience/a/brief_history.htm. Accessed 08/07/2011.

3 Reiman PR, Augustine SJ, Chao D: The action sports athlete. Sports Med Update 2007;July:2–8.

4 Schuman SH: Skateboard injuries in a campus community. Clin Pediatr 1967;6:252–254.

5 Glascoe S: The perilous skateboard. Br Med J 1977; 2:1222–1223.

6 Skateboarder Near-Death after Injury/KXAN.com. Available at: http://www.kxan.com/dpp/news/local/student-seriously-injured-skateboarding. Accessed 06/07/2011.

7 Teen Killed in Accident, Skateboarding Without a Helmet, Sherman Oaks/CA Patch. Available at: http://shermanoaks.patch.com/articles/teen-killed-in-accident-skateboarding-without-a-helmet. Accessed 06/07/2011.

8 NEISS Home. Available at: http://www.cpsc.gov/library/neiss.html. Accessed 08/07/2011.

9 Bicycling and Skating Safety Fact Sheet. Available at: http://www.safekids.org/our-work/research/fact-sheets/. Accessed 08/07/2011.

10 2010 Youth Participation in Selected Sports with Comparisons to 2001 (PDF file) – National Sporting Goods Association. Available at: http://www.nsga.org/i4a/pages/index.cfm?pageid=3494. Accessed 08/07/2011.

11 Fountain JL, Meyers MC: Skateboarding injuries. Sports Med 1996;22:360–366.

12 Kyle SB, Nance ML, Rutherford GW Jr, Winston FK: Skateboard-associated injuries: participation-based estimates and injury characteristics. J Trauma 2002; 53:686–690.

13 Zalavras C, Nikolopoulou G, Essin D, Manjra N, Zionts LE: Pediatric fractures during skateboarding, roller skating, and scooter riding. Am J Sports Med 2005;33:568–573.

14 Forsman L, Eriksson A: Skateboarding injuries of today. Br J Sports Med 2001;35:325–328.

15 Osberg JS, Schneps SE, Di Scala C, Li G: Skateboarding: more dangerous than roller skating or in-line skating. Arch Pediatr Adolesc Med 1998; 152:985–991.

16 Hawkins RW, Lyne ED: Skateboarding fractures. Am J Sports Med 1981;9:99–102.

17 Everett W: Skatepark injuries and the influence of skatepark design: a one-year consecutive case series J Emerg Med 2002;23:269–274.

18 Vaca F, Mai D, Anderson CL, Fox JC, Ferrarella N: Associated economic impact of skatepark-related injuries in Southern California. Clin Med Res 2007; 5:149–154.

19 Lustenberger T, Talving P, Barmparas G, Schnuriger B, Lam L, Inaba K, et al: Skateboard-related injuries: not to be taken lightly. A National Trauma Databank Analysis. J Trauma 2010;69:924–927.

20 Pendergrast RA Jr: Skateboard injuries in children and adolescents. J Adolesc Health Care 1990;11: 408–412.

21 Keilani M, Krall C, Lipowec L, Posch M, Komanadj TS, Crevenna R: Skateboarding injuries in Vienna: location, frequency, and severity. PM R 2010;2: 619–624.

22 Jacobs RA, Keller EL: Skateboard accidents. Pediatrics 1977;59:939–942.

23 Vaca F, Fox JC, Mai D, Anderson CL, Kwon KT, Wiechmann WF: Skatepark-related injuries in a Southern California skatepark and their associated short-term disability and healthcare utilization. Clin J Sport Med 2005;15:142–147.

24 Konkin DE, Garraway N, Hameed SM, Brown DR, Granger R, Wheeler S, et al: Population-based analysis of severe injuries from nonmotorized wheeled vehicles. Am J Surg 2006;191:615–618.
25 Illingworth CM, Jay A, Noble D, Collick M: 225 skateboard injuries in children. Clin Pediatr (Phila) 1978;17:781–782, 788–789.
26 Cass DT, Ross F: Skateboard injuries. Med J Aust 1990;153:140, 143–414.
27 Schieber RA, Olson SJ: Developing a culture of safety in a reluctant audience West J Med 2002; 176:E1–E2.
28 Finch C, Valuri G, Ozanne-Smith J: Sport and active recreation injuries in Australia: evidence from emergency department presentation./Blessures lors de la pratique d'activités sportives et d'activités physiques de loisirs en Australie: constats à partir des données présentées par les services d'urgence des hôpitaux. Br J Sports Med 1998;32:220–225.
29 Sheehan E, Mulhall KJ, Kearns S, O'Connor P, McManus F, Stephens M, et al: Impact of dedicated skate parks on the severity and incidence of skateboard- and rollerblade-related pediatric fractures. J Pediatr Orthop 2003;23:440–442.
30 Macdonald DJ, McGlone S, Exton A, Perry S: A new skatepark: the impact on the local hospital. Injury 2006;37:238–242.
31 Skateboard injuries: American Academy of Pediatrics Committee on Injury and Poison Prevention Pediatrics 1995;95:611–612.
32 Rethnam U, Yesupalan RS, Sinha A: Skateboards: are they really perilous? A retrospective study from a district hospital. BMC Res Notes 2008;1:59.
33 Skateboard Events and Competitions Calendar. Available at: http://skateboard.about.com/od/skateboardcalendar/tp/Skateboard_Events_Calendar.htm. Accessed 12/07/2011.
34 Stricker PR, Puffer JC: Renal laceration. A skateboarder's symptoms are delayed./Lésion rénale: symptômes diffères chez les pratiquants de planche à roulettes. Phys Sportsmed 1993;21:59–62, 67–68.
35 Carragher AM, Sulaiman SK, Panesar KJ: Scroto-abdominal impalement injury in a skateboard rider. J Emerg Med 1990;8:419–421.
36 Tator CH: Catastrophic Injuries in Sports and Recreation: Causes and Prevention. A Canadian Study. Toronto, University of Toronto Press, 2008.
37 Caine D, Lindner K: Preventing injury to young athletes. Part 1: Predisposing factors. Can Assoc Health Phys Educ Recreat J 1990;56:30–35.
38 Morgan WJ, Galloway DJ, Patel AR: Prevention of skateboard injuries. Scott Med J 1980;25:39–40.
39 Committee on Injury and Poison Prevention, American Academy of Pediatrics: Skateboard and scooter injuries. Pediatrics 2002;109:542–543.
40 Thompson DC, Rivara FP, Thompson RS: Effectiveness of bicycle safety helmets in preventing head injuries. JAMA 1996;276:1968.
41 Kroncke EL, Niedfeldt MW, Young CC: Use of protective equipment by adolescents in inline skating, skateboarding, and snowboarding. Clin J Sport Med 2008;18:38–43.
42 Wu BC, Oakes JM: A randomized controlled trial of sport helmet interventions in a pediatric emergency department. Pediatr Emerg Care 2005;21:730–735.

Jamie Hunter, BSc, MD
31 Lygon Road, Edinburgh EH16 5QD (UK)
Tel. +44 7752712394
E-Mail jamie.hunter@doctors.org.uk

Heggie TW, Caine DJ (eds): Epidemiology of Injury in Adventure and Extreme Sports.
Med Sport Sci. Basel, Karger, 2012, vol 58, pp 158–172

# The Epidemiology of Injury in ATV and Motocross Sports

A. Noelle Larson · Amy L. McIntosh

Division of Pediatric Orthopedic Surgery, Mayo Clinic, Rochester, Minn., USA

**Abstract**

Off-road motorsports are popular in rural and suburban areas, and allow for racing, recreation, and easy access to backcountry destinations. This chapter will review the incidence and types of injuries sustained in off-road motorsports. We completed a structured review of motocross and all-terrain vehicle (ATV) injuries, assessing for injury rates, risk factors, and mortality figures. Information for this study was obtained from a PubMed search under the terms 'motocross', 'motorcross', 'all-terrain vehicles', 'injury', 'motorcycle', 'ATV'. Abstracts and articles in the English language from 1980 onward were reviewed. Further statistics were obtained from the US Consumer Product Safety Commission publications. Operating vehicles off-road requires coordination, experience, and training. Motocross is an organized sport with national associations governing the competition of highly trained athletes. ATVs are used both recreationally and commercially, typically for farming and ranching. ATV use appears more dangerous that motocross, with a higher mortality rate, disproportionately for children. Both sports continue to have high rates of head, spinal cord, and extremity injury. Future prospective studies in off-road motorsports should evaluate the risk factors for injury and target specific areas for injury prevention. Improved training programs, use and improvement of safety helmets, and for ATV use, limiting access to minors, may improve the overall safety of off-road motorsports.



## Introduction

All-terrain vehicle (ATVs) and off-road motorcycling (motocross) are growing in popularity, for industry, recreation, and competitive sports. In the USA, the number of ATVs in use has increased from 400,000 in the 1970s to 10.5 million by 2009 [1]. In one rural US state, 30% of residents surveyed by telephone owned an ATV [2]. In rural and suburban areas, participants have access to private and public trails as well as formal courses. On the whole, injuries from off-road vehicles are increasing [1, 3, 4]. Vehicles are readily available, but substantial skill, coordination, muscle strength, and judgment are required to safely operate an off-road vehicle. This is particularly applicable to children and young adults, who may lack these psychomotor skills and are at increased risk for injury, especially as passengers. There are particular safety concerns about children operating and riding ATVs and off-road motorcycles. A growing body of literature is available on the injury patterns and severity of off-road vehicle injuries. Investigations are often prompted by the severe and disabling motocross and ATV injuries seen by emergency care providers and physicians rather than reports from coaches, riders, and team physicians. We aim to describe patterns of injuries and strategies for injury prevention for individuals participating in competitive and recreational off-road sports.

Information for this study was obtained from a PubMed search under the terms 'motocross,' 'motorcross', 'all-terrain vehicles', 'injury', 'motorcycle', and 'ATV'. Abstracts and articles in the English language from 1980 onward were reviewed. Further statistics were obtained from the US Consumer Product Safety Commission publications. Information from these national injury registries was utilized, even though the data includes both agricultural and recreational use of vehicles.

One of the authors (A.L.M.) has extensive firsthand experience developing a motocross sports medicine program and has initiated an injury-registry program. Original data from these efforts are included, particularly with respect to head injuries and motocross.

ATVs are four-wheeled motorized vehicles used extensively in rural areas for agriculture, ranching, hunting, recreation, and transportation. Vehicles may weigh from 100 to 600 lb (1 lb = 0.45 kg) and engine displacement ranges from 50 to 500 cm [3, 4]. ATVs may achieve speeds of 75 mph [5]. ATVs have a straddle seat with handlebars. In contrast, golf carts or dune buggies have steering wheels and bucket seats and are excluded from this review. In order to provide maneuverability and traction over uneven ground, ATVs have large, low inflation tires and a short wheel-based, resulting in a high center of gravity [6]. When the ATV encounters an obstacle in the path, the rider may need to adjust the steering angle, body position, and throttle almost instantaneously to avoid rollover [6]. Children and young adults may have lower body weight and may not be able to counter the rotational momentum of a vehicle by changing their center of gravity.

In most regions, ATVs are not permitted on public, paved roads and must be used in an off-road capacity. Specific regulations are dependent on jurisdiction, but for many states, there is no licensure of the driver or the vehicle. Three-wheeled ATVs were previously available, but due to vehicle instability and high injury rates, they have been taken out of production in the USA under a consent agreement between the manufacturers and the US Consumer Product Safety Commission in 1988. As part of this agreement, adult-sized vehicles were limited to riders >16 years of age [7]. Rider education programs were established, and dealers associated with the Specialty Vehicle Institute of America (SVIA) offer free training with purchase of an ATV.

Motocross is defined as use of a two-wheeled vehicle in an off-road capacity, typically for sporting or recreational purposes. The sport is increasing in popularity [8]. It is a physically demanding activity which requires endurance, coordination, and

**Table 1.** Epidemiology of ATV injuries

| Reference (first author) | Study/ setting | Years | Inclusion criteria | Patients n | Incidence | Mortality | Mean ISS (range) | Length of stay |
|---|---|---|---|---|---|---|---|---|
| Streeter 2008 [14] | National database | 2006 | all ER visits | 140,900 (estimate) | 163 ER visits per 10,000 machines in use | 1.1 deaths per 10,000 4-wheeled visits in use | n/a | n/a |
| Cvijanovich 2001 [7] | retrospective review/ estimate | 1998 | injury rate | n/a | 195 overall per 10,000 machines in use | n/a | n/a | n/a |
| Mullins 2007 [3] | retrospective state/trauma visits, includes motocross | 1998–2003 | Oregon Trauma Registry | 1,237 | 120 deaths per 1,000,000 males, 25 per 1,000,000 females | 14 (1.1%) | 10±8 | 4±5.9 |

balance. Simulated models show motocross riders spending 87–97% of their riding time above 90% of the maximum heart rate [9–11]. Sporting events at advanced levels require complex jumps and turns with vehicle heights reaching up to 10 m above the ground.

Although there is limited literature about the epidemiology, this chapter will discuss what is known about the rates and types of ATV and motocross injuries.

### Who Is Affected by Injury?

The best data regarding overall injuries rates from off-road vehicle use in the USA come from national registries. According to the National Electronic Injury Surveillance System, there were an estimated 275,123 injuries in 2006 due to ATVs, motocross, and mopeds, with 30,818 hospital admissions or deaths annually [12]. Other estimates for exclusively four-wheeled off-road vehicles show 163.0 injuries annually per 10,000 four-wheeled ATVs in use, or 1.6 injuries per 100 vehicles including all applications (table 1) [13, 14]. ATV injuries are more common in males and Caucasian individuals [15–18].

Approximately 30% of ATV injuries occur in children <16 years of age [12]. Although children only comprise 14–18% of riders, they account for 30–50% of off-road vehicle injuries [12–19]. Motocross injuries in children frequently have a high level of severity and high rates of hospitalization [20]. The American Academy of Pediatrics and American Academy of Orthopaedic Surgeons recommend against children <16 years of age riding or operating two- or four-wheeled off-road vehicles [21,

**Table 2.** ATV mortality

| Reference (first author) | Study/setting | Years | Age years | deaths n | Cause of death | Mechanism |
|---|---|---|---|---|---|---|
| Garland 2009 [1] | national database | 1982–2006 | all | 10,281 | n/a | n/a |
| Cvijanovich 2001 [7] | retrospective review, children | 1998 | n/a | 8 | 1 head injury, 7 unknown | driver (8) |
| Lister 1998 [23] | retrospective/state | 1991–1995 | n/a | 4 | n/a | n/a |
| Kirkpatrick 2007 [24] | retrospective review, level 1 trauma center, children | 2001–2007 | mean 12.5 (range 10–15) | 4 | 4 head injuries | auto collision (3), rollover (1) |

22]. Of the 4,483 children admitted for ATV accidents, the majority are male (76%), Caucasian (85%), and privately insured (63%) [19]. ATV patients aged 12–15 years have higher injury severity scores (ISS) compared to adult patients [18]. Adolescents in this age range may have an adult body size and are allowed to ride independently, but they may have not yet acquired the appropriate psychomotor skills and cognitive skills to operate a motor vehicle [18].

In the USA from 1982 to 2008, there have been 10,281 ATV-related deaths (table 2) [1, 23, 24]. A 1999–2007 summary report estimates 0.9–1.4 deaths annually per 10,000 vehicles in use [1]. Of those, 26% of deaths were in children <16 years and 12% in children <12 years [1]. For an average ATV user, age 30 with 8 years of driving experience who rides a 300-$cm^3$ engine recreationally 23 h/month, the average risk of injury is 0.25% per year [4].

In adult competitive motocross riders, reports have shown injury rates ranging from 2.7 to 29.2 per 1,000 h of riding (table 3) [25–27]. This represents up to 4.5 injuries per race [25]. In one study, motocross racing had a significantly higher injury rate compared to trial racing, which involves a single participant negotiating complex terrain at low speeds [27]. Motocross injuries are more frequent in insured, male and Caucasian individuals [16].

### Where Does Injury Occur?

#### *Anatomic Location*

Knowledge of the anatomical location of injury can be vital for sports medicine staff as well as epidemiologists, helping to highlight which areas are more likely to be injured and to assist with directions of preventive research. For ATV injuries, the

**Table 3.** Motocross injuries and severity

| Reference (first author) | Study/setting | Race days n (years) | Injuries, (number/riders) | Mean ISS (range) | Injuries/1,000 exposure hours |
|---|---|---|---|---|---|
| Colburn 2003 [26] | prospective/adult competition | 24 (1992–1995) | 9.6% (172/1,787) | 3.9 (1–34) | 2.7 |
| Gobbi 2004 [25] | retrospective/ adult competition | n/a (1980–1991) | 9.5% (1,500 injuries/ 15,870) | n/a | 22.7 |
| Tomida 2005 [27] | retrospective questionnaire/ adults | n/a (3/2001–6/2002) | 53% (32/60) | n/a | 49.2 |

head and extremities are the most frequently injured anatomic area (table 4) [4, 17, 28]. In a series of 208 patients at two level 1 trauma centers, 26% had major head injuries (coma or intracranial hemorrhage) and an additional 15% had concussions or loss of consciousness [18]. A prospective series of 193 patients reported that 47% of patients sustained a head injury [28]. Of the 208 patients, 23% had extremity injuries and 14.9% had spinal fractures, 4 patients (1.9%) with a neurologic deficit. A similar trend has been seen in children as well (fig. 1). Of the 4,483 children admitted for ATV injuries in 2006, 7.4% had spinal fractures [19]. Of those with spine injuries, polytrauma was common, with a mean of 4.3 injuries per pediatric patient [19].

Head injuries are also the most commonly reported cause of death in ATV accidents, followed by exsanguination from great vessel or internal organ injury [2, 18, 29]. Laryngotracheal trauma may also occur from encountering unseen wire fences at high speeds [1]. Deaths have also been associated with racing, jumping, rollover accidents, and alcohol use [30].

Motocross patients typically present with musculoskeletal injuries and/or head trauma. Up to half of patients present with extremity trauma [16, 20, 26]. The most common fractures in the pediatric population are forearm, clavicle, tibia, and femur (fig. 2) [16, 20]. Left-sided injuries are more frequent, perhaps due to the location of foot-operated gear shifts [25]. Series have reported that 30–36% of pediatric patients presenting with a motocross injury require surgery, typically orthopedic procedures (fig. 3) [16, 20]. Tibial plateau and talus fractures have also been reported in adults participating in competitive motocross [25, 31, 32]. Upper extremity fractures are common as well. One series reports that up to 20% of distal radius fractures occur simply from the impact of landing through the handlebars, due to improper regulations of the forward suspension of the motorcycle. The crash then occurs after the fracture, due to loss of control of the vehicle [25].

**Table 4.** ATV injuries

| Reference (first author) | Study/setting | Years | Inclusion criteria | Patients n | Mechanism | Injuries | Mean ISS (range) | Positive ethanol screen | Mean length of stay days |
|---|---|---|---|---|---|---|---|---|---|
| Alawi 2006 [30] | retrospective/ regional/ children | 1998–2003 | age <18 ISS ≥12 | 17 (1.6% of pediatric trauma patients) | 17 rollover | internal 8 head 6 fracture 13 | 22.8 (1–34) | n/a | 9.7 |
| Smith 2005 [18] | Retrospective/ 2 Level 1 Trauma Centers | 1994–2003 | all admissions | 208 | 57 rollover 55 ejected 62 other/ collision | internal 75 head 86 fracture 83 | 12.3 | n/a | n/a |
| Kirkpatrick 2007 [24] | retrospective review, level 1 trauma center | 2001–2006 | trauma registry, age <16 | 73 | n/a | head 33 facial 20 fracture 36 | 10.3 | n/a | n/a |
| Lister 1998 [23] | retrospective/ state | 1991–1995 | age <16 | 218 | n/a | head 88 facial 77 internal 98 fracture 116 | 8.8±6.0 | 1% | 4.3 |
| Brown 2002 [15] | retrospective/ level 1 trauma center | 2006 | age <18 | 109 | 17 rollover 45 ejected 40 other | head/ neck 22 internal 16 fracture 25 | 8.3±7.2 | n/a | 6.3 ± 13.9 |
| Cvijanovich 2001 [7] | retrospective/ state | 1992–1996 | age <16, admissions | 130 | n/a | head/neck 31 internal 20 fracture 52 | 8±6.0 | n/a | 2 (median) |
| Mullins 2007 [3] | retrospective/ level 1 trauma center | 1998–2005 | all ATV trauma admissions | 197 | n/a | head/neck 91 internal 105 fracture 76 | 14±10.3 | 14% | 8±9.5 |

Motocross patients with chest trauma typically present with other associated injuries [16]. Rare catastrophic injuries have been reported, including aortic false aneurysm and cardiac ischemia due to coronary artery dissection from blunt chest trauma [33, 34]. Spine injuries with permanent neurologic defect have been reported, despite the use of safety equipment (table 5) [25]. In one series, 9% of patients presented with a spine fracture (fig. 4) [16].

In motocross, head injuries are also very common. Head injury and concussions are commonly sustained in motocross riders, with 22–33% of pediatric patients

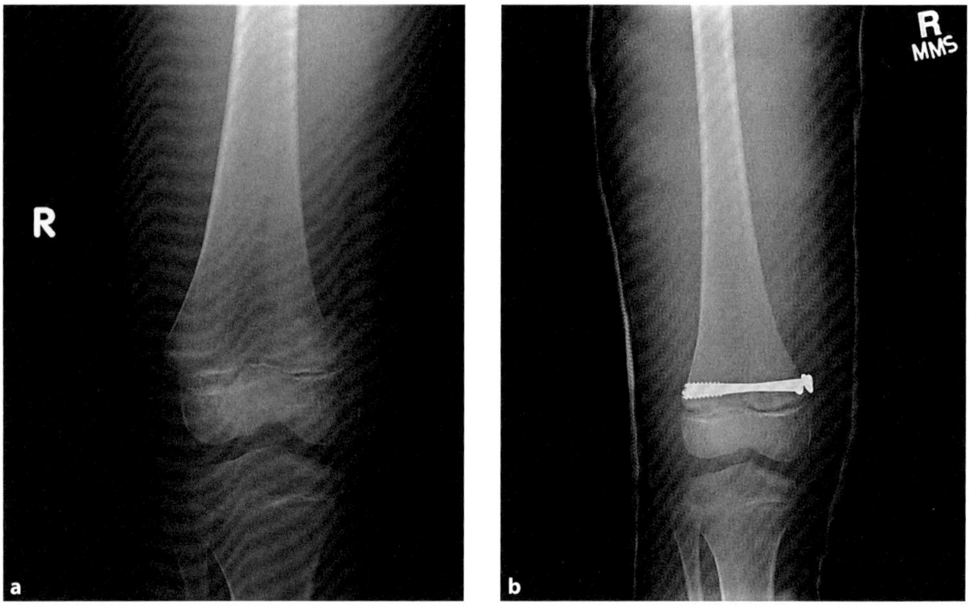


**Fig. 1.** **a** Radiograph of a distal femoral fracture involving the growth plate in a 7-year-old female who was operating a four-wheeled vehicle when she struck a stationary plow. **b** Radiograph following surgical fixation of the fracture with screw placement. Her risk of growth plate arrest resulting in an angular deformity or cessation of growth at the femur nears 50%.

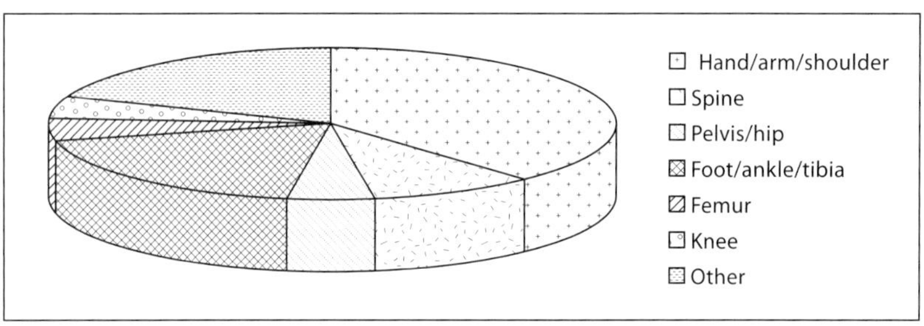


**Fig. 2.** Distribution of orthopedic injuries in children due to motocross [19].

presenting with head injury [16, 20]. In a prospective survey of 127 motocross riders, 50% reported sustaining a concussion during that season. The majority suspended participation following their injury for a mean of 2.7 weeks. Concussive symptoms included memory problems, photophobia, headaches, nausea/vomiting. In the pediatric population, many participants will not present for medical care following minor concussion, with up to 30.1% of surveyed riders continuing to compete despite symptoms of a concussion [35]. A history of multiple concussions was reported by 36% of the riders [35]. These are concerning figures with the new awareness of long-

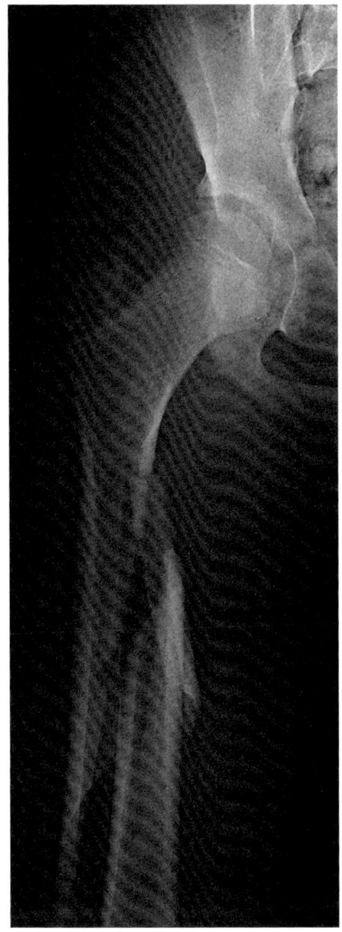

**Fig. 3.** High-energy, comminuted femur fracture in an 8-year-old motocross participant. Surgical fixation is required for this fracture pattern.

term sequelae of repetitive head trauma [36–38]. In other sports, chronic traumatic encephalopathy of the brain have been seen on autopsy in soccer or football players as young as 23 years who have a history of repetitive minor neurotrauma [36, 37]. Major head injuries such as intracerebral hemorrhage, skull fracture, or subarachnoid hemorrhage are less frequent, but have been documented in 1–5% of motocross patients, despite the use of helmets [16–20].

*Environmental Location*

Reports on the location of injury are limited. One case-controlled study found a higher rate of ATV injuries with recreational versus occupational use [4]. The US states with the highest reported numbers of ATV deaths are California, Pennsylvania, and Texas [1].

One report of elite motocross riders in Japan found a higher rate of motocross injuries during practice than during competition, perhaps because during the practice

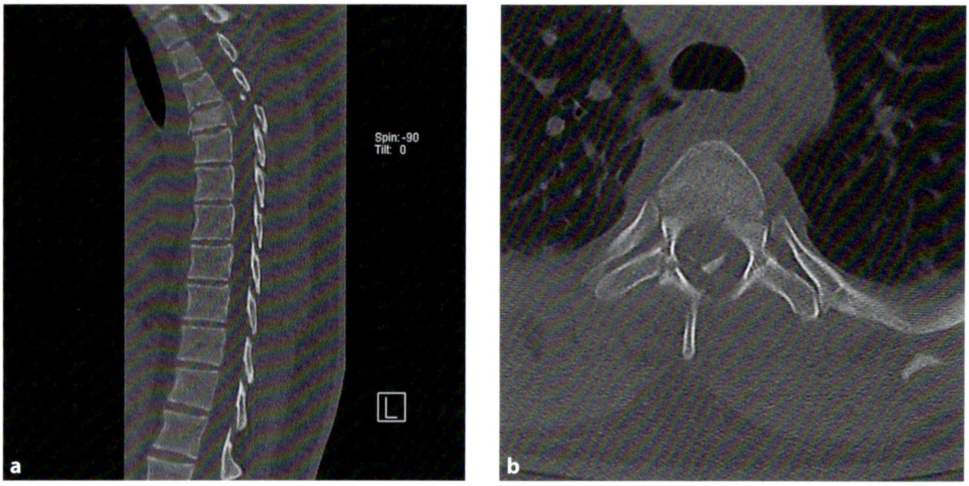


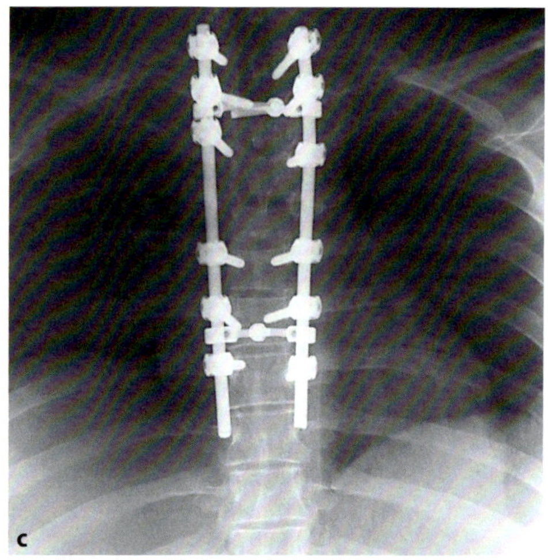


**Fig. 4. a** Sagittal CT image of the thoracic spine in a 17-year-old male who sustained a T4 burst fracture when he fell from his motorbike during a competition and was struck by another rider. **b** Axial view shows vertebral fragments in the spinal canal with compression of the spinal cord. **c** The canal was decompressed and the spine was stabilized with rods and pedicle screws. The patient remained neurologically intact throughout treatment.

**Table 5.** Distribution of motocross injuries

| Reference (first author) | Total number of injury episodes/setting | Fractures | Spine fractures | Permanent neurologic sequelae, n | Head injuries |
|---|---|---|---|---|---|
| Colburn 2003 [26] | 172 (adult competition) | 49 | 1 | 0 | 21 |
| Gobbi 2004 [25] | 1,500 (adult competition) | 450 | 26 | 8 (5 paraplegia, 3 tetraplegia) | 86 |
| Tomida 2005 [27] | 32 (adult competition) | 26 | 1 | 0 | n/a |
| Larson 2009 [20] | 299 (pediatric competition) | 217 | 13 | 2 (residual weakness after spinal cord injury, partial hemiparesis after head injury) | 55 |

rounds riders compete aggressively to obtain a good starting position [27]. The same report noted the majority of accidents occurred on curves, bumps, and steep slopes [27]. A report on pediatric motocross injuries found the majority of patients presenting for medical evaluation sustained the injury at a formal course, but this study was unable to differentiate practice rounds from races [20]. A comparison of stadium versus outdoor motocross competition found a much higher rate of injuries, including permanent paralysis, during the indoor events [25].

## When Does Injury Occur?

*Injury Onset*

Most motocross and ATV injuries are acute, although chronic exertional compartment syndrome of the forearm has been reported in a motocross patient [39]. Commonly called, 'arm pump,' riders complain about tightness in the forearms and weakness in the hands, which is attributed to loss of control of the vehicle [8]. This is thought to be a type of chronic exertional compartment syndrome, but also may be associated with deconditioning, tight grip on the handlebars, or dehydration [8]. Little is known about chronic injuries in motocross and ATV patients.

*Chronometry (Time into Practice, Time of Day, Season)*

There is some evidence that night-time use of off-road vehicles is a risk factor for injury, as is driving the vehicle on highways or in traffic with conventional vehicles. Accidents typically occur when the vehicle rolls over or strikes a stationery object.

In our limited series, we found several motocross riders injured during their first attempts at riding, although there is limited epidemiologic data to confirm these findings [20]. In data from adult competitors, injuries appear to be evenly distributed across multi-day events [26].

## What Is the Outcome?

*Injury Type*

The distribution of injuries by type may not be truly reflective of the percent distribution of injury types actually experienced. Since these are injuries most often presented to emergency departments of hospitals, they are likely to be more severe in nature.

Orthopedic and trauma brain injuries are most common following motocross and ATV injuries. In children, reported neurologic injuries after motocross accidents have shown some improvement with time [20]. Reported paraplegia and tetraplegia following motocross accidents in adults have resulted in permanent disability and impairment [25].

*Injury Severity*
In a series of 270 patients with motocross injuries treated over a 1-year period at a trauma center, the mean ISS was 6.8 (range 1–38) [16]. Mean ISS from professional competition, including patients who only sought medical attention onsite at the race track, was 3.9 (range 1–34) [26]. Two retrospective series found that surgery was required in more than one third of patients with motocross injuries [16, 20].

On the whole, injury severity is higher in ATV accidents. Mean ISS from ATV accidents ranges from 9.2 to 13.6 (table 3) [1, 3, 17, 18, 28, 29]. Mean length of hospital stay ranges from 4.0 to 8.75 days [3, 17, 29].

*Clinical Outcome*
Mortality rates of ATV riders presenting for treatment range from 0.0 to 1.0% [3]. Little is known about the long-term outcomes of ATV injuries, such as rates of post-traumatic arthritis, sequelae of head injuries, and other trauma.

Many motocross participants return to play quickly after their injury. Over time, the typical motocross athlete has multiple injury episodes [20]. In the case of head injuries, this is concerning, given the recent data about the long-term effects of repetitive head injuries in football and boxing [37, 38]. In one series of pediatric patients with motocross injures, there was a patient who sustained a spinal cord injury, who had nearly full recovery and one patient with hemiplegia following a head injury with partial recovery [20]. Neither patient returned to motocross.

*Economic Effects*
Mean billed charges at hospitalization for a pediatric ATV injury in 1996 was estimated at USD 4,240 [7]. Mean billed charges of pediatric motocross injury in 2000 was estimated at USD 14,947 [20]. Including quality-of-life measures, wages, and medical services, the estimated cost of an ATV fatality is USD 3.0 million [2]. The estimated total cost of ATV injuries by the Consumer Product Safety Commission is USD 6.5 billion [6].

## What Are the Risk Factors?

A case-control study evaluating risk factors for ATV injuries reported the highest risk for injury in children <16 years old [4]. Risk of injury decreased with more hours of driving experience, nonrecreational activities, and smaller engine size [4]. A 1% increase in driving experience reduced the risk of injury by 0.4%, and a 1% decrease in engine size increased risk of injury by 0.9% [4]. In one report of 112 ATV deaths, alcohol was detected in the blood of 50% of ATV victims and illicit substances in 21% of the decedents [40].

Motocross has limited data on the risk factors for injury. As has been classically reported in other sports, laboratory and field studies have shown improved coordination and outcome in motocross skills later in the day, with a diurnal effect noted [41, 42]. Thus, there may be increased risk of injury earlier in the day, although this is not proven. A report of injuries sustained at national competitions showed no association between rider experience and risk of injury [27].

### What Are the Inciting Events?

Typically, ATV accidents occur when the vehicle hits a stationary object, a rider falls from the vehicle, or the vehicle rolls over [15, 18, 28]. ATV riders are more likely to collide with a stationary object than a moving object [18]. Collisions with stationery objects are more frequent injury mechanisms among children [28]. Collision with another vehicle is relatively rare and represents only a fracture of the injuries [29]. Children are frequently injured when riding as passengers or when driving an adult-sized vehicle [15]. From 16 to 63% of ATV accidents are reported to include a rollover mechanism [15, 28]. Only half of the rollover accidents involved riding on a slope, and the remainder occurred on flat or uneven ground [28]. Backward rollovers are associated with traveling up a slope [28]. ATV rollover accidents have been associated with a higher level of injury severity, with the vehicle frequently landing on the patient [28]. Of the pediatric patients presenting to one center with an ISS >12, all were victims of rollover accidents [30].

Studies from adult motocross racing show common injury mechanisms include hitting a stationery object/single vehicle accidents (70% of accidents) [26, 27]. Other causes include loss of traction and collision with another vehicle [26]. Ejection from the handlebars is associated with striking an object and upper extremity fractures [26].

### Injury Prevention

There is conflicting evidence for the benefit of helmet use in ATV trauma. One study showed associated lower rates of traumatic brain injury, death, and neck/facial injuries with helmet use [43], while other studies have shown no difference in ISS between helmeted and unhelmeted riders [17]. The Consumer Product Safety Commission suggests that the death rate would fall with the use of mandatory helmets. Safety training is offered with the purchase of every vehicle. Further the Consumer Product Safety Commission recommends participating in free training sessions upon purchase of the vehicle. Unfortunately, <10% of purchasers opt to participate in the free safety training [6].

The American Academy of Orthopaedic Surgeons has made the following recommendations with regard to ATVs: (1) read the operator manual; (2) take a training course; (3) never carry a passenger; (4) never operate the vehicle on paved or public roads; (5) wear safety equipment, including helmet and eye protection; (6) never consume alcohol prior to operating a vehicle; (7) never attempt jumps or stunts; (8) use the vehicle at low speeds; (9) do not allow children <18 to drive or ride the vehicle; (10) never lend your vehicle to others; (11) never operate your vehicle after dark, and (12) always use headlights [22]. There is little evidence to support these recommendations but given the high rate of injuries, these are reasonable measures.

There are limited data about the use of safety equipment in motocross, since most competitive settings require the full protective equipment, including eye, trunk, knee protection, as well as boots, helmets, and gloves. Open-face helmets ('jet-type') have a higher associated rate of facial laceration and trauma due to limited protection from flying debris [25]. Specialized neck braces are available, but have not been shown to decrease the rate of cervical spine injury [8].

Safety at the motocross site requires advanced planning. Spectator-free areas should be designated, with access points for medical personnel [8]. Transportation to a hospital should be prearranged and available the site. Flaggers should identify injured competitors and stop the race or redirect traffic. Injuries often occur in areas that are hidden from the view of oncoming racers. Rescuers should proceed only to a safe scene. C-spine precautions and ABCs of trauma should be initiated. Any patient with signs of a concussion or loss of consciousness should be transported to a medical care facility [8].

## Further Research

Significant work remains to be done on injury epidemiology and prevention in these two relatively new sports. Clearly, there is significant economic and social cost to injuries sustained from motocross and ATV competition. Participants are avid about their sport, and these often represent family events, with parents and children riding together. Further work is necessary to determine the risk factors for injury and to implement preventative measures to improve the safety of the sport.

## References


1 Garland S: 2009 Annual Report of ATV-Related Deaths and Injuries. Consumer Product Safety Commission, 2010.

2 Helmkamp JC: Family fun-family tragedy: ATV-related deaths involving family members. Inj Prev 2007;13:426–428.

3 Mullins RJ, Brand D, Lenfesty B, Newgard CD, Hedges JR, Ham B: Statewide assessment of injury and death rates among riders of off-road vehicles treated at trauma centers. J Am Coll Surg 2007;204:216–224.

4 Rodgers GB, Adler P: Risk factors for all-terrain vehicle injuries: a national case-control study. Am J Epidemiol 2001;153:1112–1118.

5 Rodgers GB: All-terrain vehicle injury risks and the effects of regulation. Accid Anal Prev 1993;25:335–346.

6 Scutchfield SB: All-terrain vehicles: injuries and prevention. Clin Orthop Relat Res 2003:61–72.

7 Cvijanovich NZ, Cook LJ, Mann NC, Dean JM: A population-based assessment of pediatric all-terrain vehicle injuries. Pediatrics 2001;108:631–635.

8 Grange JT, Bodnar JA, Corbett SW: Motocross medicine. Curr Sports Med Rep 2009;8:125–130.
9 Ascensao A, Azevedo V, Ferreira R, Oliveira E, Marques F, Magalhaes J: Physiological, biochemical and functional changes induced by a simulated 30 min off-road competitive motocross heat. J Sports Med Phys Fitness 2008;48:311–319.
10 Konttinen T, Kyrolainen H, Hakkinen K: Cardiorespiratory and neuromuscular responses to motocross riding. J Strength Cond Res 2008;22:202–209.
11 Konttinen T, Hakkinen K, Kyrolainen H: Cardiopulmonary loading in motocross riding. J Sports Sci 2007;25:995–999.
12 National Electronic Injury Surveillance System Data Highlights – 2006. Consumer Product Safety Review 2007;11:2–6.
13 2005 ATV Annual Report; in Commission USCPS (ed). Consumer Product Safety Review 2007:5–7.
14 Streeter R: 2006 Annual Report of ATV-Related Deaths and Injuries. United States of America. Consumer Product Safety Commission, 2008.
15 Brown RL, Koepplinger ME, Mehlman CT, Gittelman M, Garcia VF: All-terrain vehicle and bicycle crashes in children: epidemiology and comparison of injury severity. J Pediatr Surg 2002;37:375–380.
16 Gorski TF, Gorski YC, McLeod G, et al: Patterns of injury and outcomes associated with motocross accidents. Am Surg 2003;69:895–898.
17 Gittelman MA, Pomerantz WJ, Groner JI, Smith GA: Pediatric all-terrain vehicle-related injuries in Ohio from 1995 to 2001: using the injury severity score to determine whether helmets are a solution. Pediatrics 2006;117:2190–2195.
18 Smith LM, Pittman MA, Marr AB, et al: Unsafe at any age: a retrospective review of all-terrain vehicle injuries in two level I trauma centers from 1995 to 2003. J Trauma 2005;58:783–788.
19 Sawyer JR, Bernard MS, Schroeder RJ, Kelly DM, Warnersurname WC Jr: Trends in all-terrain vehicle-related spinal injuries in children and adolescents. J Pediatr Orthop 2011;31:623–627.
20 Larson AN, Stans AA, Shaughnessy WJ, Dekutoski MB, Quinn MJ, McIntosh AL: Motocross morbidity: economic cost and injury distribution in children. J Pediatr Orthop 2009;29:847–850.
21 All-terrain vehicle injury prevention: two-, three-, and four-wheeled unlicensed motor vehicles. Pediatrics 2000;105:1352–1354.
22 American Academy of Orthopaedic Surgeons: Position statement: all-terrain vehicles. Available at http://www.aaos.org/about/papers/position/1101/asp. Accessed August 1, 2011.
23 Lister DG, Carl J 3rd, Morgan JH 3rd, et al: Pediatric all-terrain vehicle trauma: a 5-year statewide experience. J Pediatr Surg 1998;33:1081–1083.
24 Kirkpatrick R, Puffinbarger W, Sullivan JA: All-terrain vehicle injuries in children. J Pediatr Orthop 2007;27:725–728.
25 Gobbi A, Tuy B, Panuncialman I: The incidence of motocross injuries: a 12-year investigation. Knee Surg Sports Traumatol Arthrosc 2004;12:574–580.
26 Colburn NT, Meyer RD: Sports injury or trauma? Injuries of the competition off-road motorcyclist. Injury 2003;34:207–214.
27 Tomida Y, Hirata H, Fukuda A, et al: Injuries in elite motorcycle racing in Japan. Br J Sports Med 2005;39:508–511.
28 Brandenburg MA, Brown SJ, Archer P, Brandt EN Jr: All-terrain vehicle crash factors and associated injuries in patients presenting to a regional trauma center. J Trauma 2007;63:994–999.
29 Lynch JM, Gardner MJ, Worsey J: The continuing problem of all-terrain vehicle injuries in children. J Pediatr Surg 1998;33:329–332.
30 Alawi K, Lynch T, Lim R: All-terrain vehicle major injury patterns in children: a five-year review in Southwestern Ontario. CJEM 2006;8:277–280.
31 Barnett TM, Teasdall RD: Bilateral lateral process fracture of the talus in a motocross rider. Foot Ankle Int 2008;29:245–247.
32 White SL, Harpaz NT, Jolly GP, Gorecki GA: High-energy bilateral talar neck fractures secondary to motocross injury. J Foot Ankle Surg 1999;38:214–218.
33 Burns BJ, Healy G: Coronary artery dissection: an unusual cause of hypoxia in blunt trauma. Prehosp Emerg Care 2011;15:414–417.
34 Bizzarri F, Mattia C, Ricci M, et al: Traumatic aortic arch false aneurysm after blunt chest trauma in a motocross rider. J Cardiothorac Surg 2008;3:23.
35 McIntosh AL: Concussive injuries in pediatric motocross riders: a prospective observational study. Rochester, Mayo Clinic, 2011.
36 Halstead ME, Walter KD: American Academy of Pediatrics. Clinical report – sport-related concussion in children and adolescents. Pediatrics 2010;126:597–615.
37 McKee AC, Cantu RC, Nowinski CJ, et al: Chronic traumatic encephalopathy in athletes: progressive tauopathy after repetitive head injury. J Neuropathol Exp Neurol 2009;68:709–735.
38 McCrea M, Guskiewicz KM, Marshall SW, et al: Acute effects and recovery time following concussion in collegiate football players: the NCAA Concussion Study. JAMA 2003;290:2556–2563.
39 Gielen JL, Peersman B, Peersman G, et al: Chronic exertional compartment syndrome of the forearm in motocross racers: findings on MRI. Skeletal Radiol 2009;38:1153–1161.

40 Hall AJ, Bixler D, Helmkamp JC, Kraner JC, Kaplan JA: Fatal all-terrain vehicle crashes: injury types and alcohol use. Am J Prev Med 2009;36:311–316.
41 Bougard C, Davenne D: Effects of sleep deprivation and time-of-day on selected physical abilities in off-road motorcycle riders. Eur J Appl Physiol 2012;112: 59–67.
42 Bougard C, Moussay S, Davenne D: An assessment of the relevance of laboratory and motorcycling tests for investigating time of day and sleep deprivation influences on motorcycling performance. Accid Anal Prev 2008;40:635–643.
43 Bowman SM, Aitken ME, Helmkamp JC, Maham SA, Graham CJ: Impact of helmets on injuries to riders of all-terrain vehicles. Inj Prev 2009;15:3–7.

A. Noelle Larson, MD, Assist. Prof.
Division of Pediatric Orthopedic Surgery, Mayo Clinic
200 1st St SW, Rochester, MN 55905 (USA)
Tel. +1 507 284 2995
E-Mail larson.noelle@mayo.edu

# Author Index

# Subject Index